BETWEEN TWO KINGDOMS

BETWEEN TWO KINGDOMS

what almost dying taught me about living

Suleika Jaouad

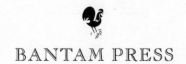

BANTAM PRESS

TRANSWORLD PUBLISHERS
Penguin Random House, One Embassy Gardens,
8 Viaduct Gardens, London SW11 7BW
www.penguin.co.uk

Transworld is part of the Penguin Random House group of companies
whose addresses can be found at global.penguinrandomhouse.com

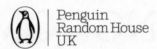

Penguin
Random House
UK

First published in Great Britain in 2021 by Bantam Press
an imprint of Transworld Publishers

Copyright © Suleika Jaouad 2021
Map by Nick Springer copyright © 2021 by Springer Cartographics LLC

Suleika Jaouad has asserted her right under the Copyright,
Designs and Patents Act 1988 to be identified as the author of this work.

A CIP catalogue record for this book
is available from the British Library.

ISBNs
9781787632318 (hb)
9781787630512 (tpb)

Printed and bound in Great Britain by Clays Ltd, Elcograf S.p.A.

The authorized representative in the EEA is Penguin Random House Ireland,
Morrison Chambers, 32 Nassau Street, Dublin D02 YH68.

Penguin Random House is committed to a sustainable
future for our business, our readers and our planet. This book
is made from Forest Stewardship Council® certified paper.

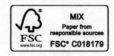

For Melissa Carroll and Max Ritvo—the ink behind it all.

And for all the others who crossed the river too soon.

Until death, it is all life.

—MIGUEL DE CERVANTES

CONTENTS

CONTENTS

AUTHOR'S NOTE

TO WRITE THIS BOOK, I relied upon my journals, my medical records, and interviews I conducted with many of the people who appear in the story, as well as my own memory. I've also included excerpts of letters, some of which have been lightly edited for the sake of brevity.

To preserve the anonymity of certain individuals, I modified identifying details and changed the following names, listed in alphabetical order: Dennis, Estelle, Jake, Joanie, Karen, Sean, and Will.

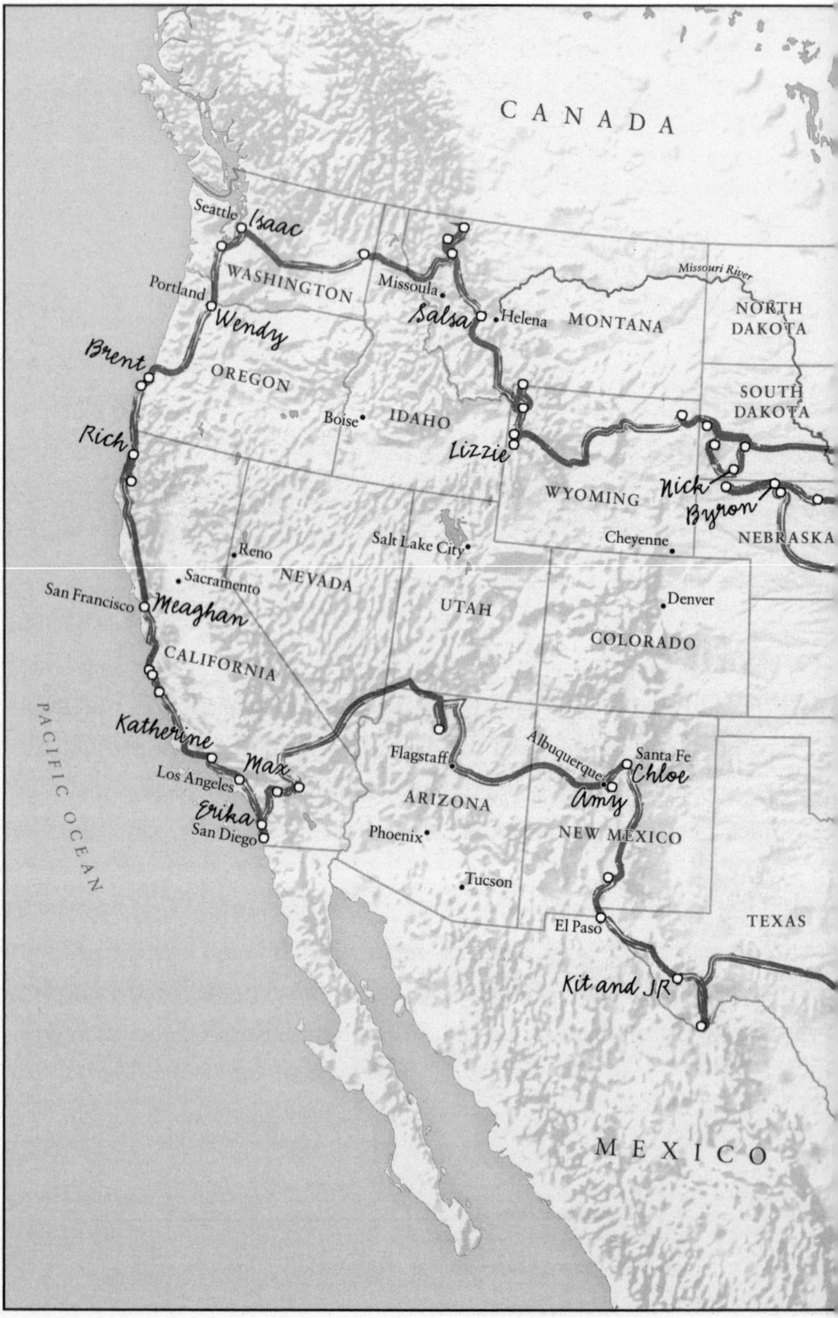
CANADA
Seattle
Isaac
WASHINGTON
Portland
Wendy
Missoula
Salsa
Helena
MONTANA
Missouri River
NORTH DAKOTA
Brent
OREGON
SOUTH DAKOTA
Boise
IDAHO
Lizzie
Rich
WYOMING
Nick
Byron
Salt Lake City
Cheyenne
NEBRASKA
Reno
Sacramento
NEVADA
San Francisco
Meaghan
UTAH
Denver
COLORADO
CALIFORNIA
PACIFIC OCEAN
Katherine
Max
Flagstaff
Albuquerque
Santa Fe
Chloe
Los Angeles
ARIZONA
Amy
Erika
San Diego
Phoenix
NEW MEXICO
Tucson
El Paso
TEXAS
Kit and JR
MEXICO

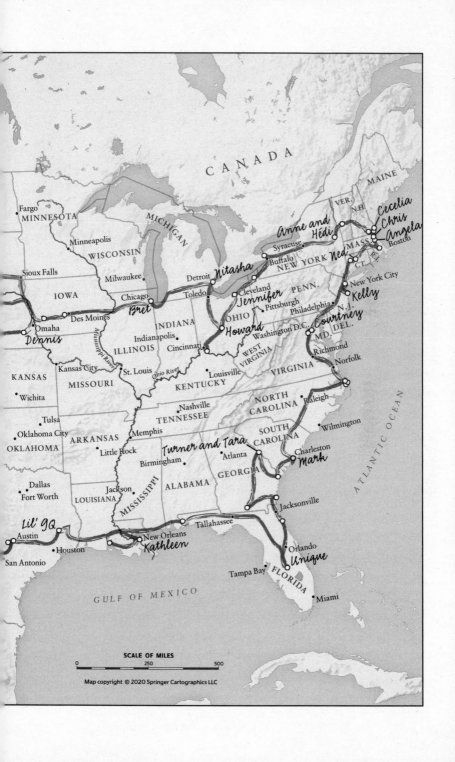

PART
ONE

1

THE ITCH

IT BEGAN WITH an itch. Not a metaphorical itch to travel the world or some quarter-life crisis, but a literal, physical itch. A maddening, claw-at-your-skin, keep-you-up-at-night itch that surfaced during my senior year of college, first on the tops of my feet and then moving up my calves and thighs. I tried to resist scratching, but the itch was relentless, spreading across the surface of my skin like a thousand invisible mosquito bites. Without realizing what I was doing, my hand began meandering down my legs, my nails raking my jeans in search of relief, before burrowing under the hem to sink directly into flesh. I itched during my part-time job at the campus film lab. I itched under the big wooden desk of my library carrel. I itched while dancing with friends on the beer-slicked floors of basement taprooms. I itched while I slept. A scree of oozing nicks, thick scabs, and fresh scars soon marred my legs as if they had been beaten with rose thistles. Bloody harbingers of a mounting struggle taking place inside of me.

"It might be a parasite you picked up while studying abroad," a Chinese herbalist told me before sending me off with foul-smelling supplements and bitter teas. A nurse at the college health center thought it might be eczema and recommended a cream. A general practitioner surmised that it was stress-related and gave me samples of an antianxiety medication. But no one seemed to know for sure, so I tried not to make a big deal out of it. I hoped it would clear up on its own.

Every morning, I would crack the door of my dorm room, scan the hall, and sprint in my towel to the communal bathroom before anyone could see my limbs. I washed my skin with a wet cloth, watching the crimson streaks swirl down the shower drain. I slathered myself in drugstore potions made of witch hazel tonic and I plugged my nose as I drank the bitter tea concoctions. Once the weather turned too warm to wear jeans every day, I invested in a collection of opaque black tights. I purchased dark-colored sheets to mask the rusty stains. And when I had sex, I had sex with the lights off.

Along with the itch came the naps. The naps that lasted two, then four, then six hours. No amount of sleep seemed to appease my body. I began dozing through orchestra rehearsals and job interviews, deadlines and dinner, only to wake up feeling even more depleted. "I've never felt so tired in my life," I confessed to my friends one day, as we were walking to class. "Me too, me too," they commiserated. Everyone was tired. We'd witnessed more sunrises in the last semester than we had in our entire lives, a combination of logging long hours at the library to finish our senior theses followed by boozy parties that raged until dawn. I lived at the heart of the Princeton campus, on the top floor of a Gothic-style dorm, crested with turrets and grimacing gargoyles. At the end of yet another late night, my friends would congregate in my room for one last nightcap. My room had big cathedral windows and we liked to sit on the sills with our legs dangling over the edge, watching as drunken revelers stumbled home and the first amber rays streaked the stone-paved courtyard. Graduation was on the horizon, and we were determined to savor these final weeks together before we all scattered, even if that meant pushing our bodies to their limits.

And yet, I worried my fatigue was different.

Alone in my bed, after everyone had gone, I sensed a feasting taking place under my skin, something wending its way through my arteries, gnawing at my sanity. As my energy evaporated and the itch intensified, I told myself it was because the parasite's appetite was growing. But deep down, I doubted there ever was a parasite. I began to wonder if the real problem was me.

In the months that followed, I felt at sea, close to sinking, grasping at anything that might buoy me. For a while I managed. I graduated, then joined my classmates in the mass exodus to New York City. I found an ad on Craigslist for a spare bedroom in a large, floor-through loft located above an art supply store on Canal Street. It was the summer of 2010 and a heat wave had sucked the oxygen out of the city. As I emerged from the subway, the stench of festering garbage smacked me in the face. Commuters and hordes of tourists shopping for knockoff designer bags jostled each other on the sidewalks. The apartment was a third-floor walk-up and by the time I lugged my suitcase to the front door, sweat had turned my white tank top see-through. I introduced myself to my new roommates; there were nine of them. They were all in their twenties and aspiring something-or-others: three actors, two models, a chef, a jewelry designer, a graduate student, and a financial analyst. Eight hundred dollars a month bought each of us our own windowless cave partitioned by paper-thin drywall that a slumlord had erected to get the most bang for his buck.

I had scored a summer internship at the Center for Constitutional Rights, and when I showed up on my first day, I felt awed to be in the same room as some of the most fearless civil liberties lawyers in the country. The work felt important, but the internship was unpaid and living in New York City was like walking around with a giant hole in my wallet. I quickly blew through the two thousand dollars I'd saved up over the school year. Even with the babysitting and restaurant jobs I worked in the evenings, I was barely scraping by.

Imagining my future—expansive yet empty—filled me with terror. In moments when I allowed myself to daydream, it thrilled me, too. The possibilities of who I might become and where I might land felt infinite, a spool of ribbon unfurling far beyond what my mind's eye could see. I envisioned a career as a foreign correspondent in North Africa, where my dad is from and where I'd lived for a stint as a kid. I also toyed with the idea of law school, which seemed like a more prudent route. Frankly, I needed money. I had only been able to attend an Ivy League college because I'd received a full scholarship. But out here, in the real world, I didn't have the same kind of safety nets—trust funds, family connections, six-figure jobs on Wall Street—as many of my classmates.

It was easier to fret about the uncertainty ahead than to confront another, even more unsettling shift. During my last semester, to combat the fatigue, I had chugged caffeinated energy drinks. When those stopped working, a boy I'd briefly dated gave me some of his Adderall to survive finals. But soon that wasn't enough either. Cocaine was a party staple in my circle of friends, and there were always guys hanging around who offered a line here and there for free. Nobody batted an eye when I started partaking. My roommates in the Canal Street loft had turned out to be hard-partying types, too. I began to take uppers the way some people add an extra shot of espresso to their coffee—a means to an end, a way to stave off my deepening exhaustion. In my journal, I wrote: *Stay afloat.*

By the last days of summer, I struggled to recognize myself. The muffled sound of my alarm clock dragged like a dull knife through dreamless sleep. Each morning, I'd stumble out of bed and stand in front of the floor-length mirror, taking inventory of the damage. Scratches and streaks of drying blood covered my legs in new places. My hair hung to my waist in dull, chaotic waves that I was too tired to brush. Shadowy crescents deepened into dark moons under big bloodshot eyes. Too burned-out to face sunlight, I started showing up later and later to my internship; then, one day, I stopped showing up altogether.

I disliked the person I was becoming—a person who tumbled headfirst into each day, in constant motion but without any sense of direction; a person who reconstructed blackouts, night after night, like some private investigator; a person who constantly reneged on commitments; a person who was too embarrassed to pick up her parents' phone calls. *This isn't me,* I thought, staring at my reflection with disgust. I needed to clean up my act. I needed to find a real job, one that paid. I needed some distance from my college crew and my Canal Street roommates. I needed to get the hell out of New York City, and soon.

On an August morning, a few days after I quit the internship, I rose early and took my laptop out to the fire escape and started searching for jobs. It had been a rainless summer, and the sun blazed, baking my skin to a tan, leaving little white dots like braille all over my legs where the scratching had scarred. A position for a paralegal at an American law firm in Paris caught my eye, and on a whim I decided to apply. I spent all day working on my cover letter. I made sure to mention that French was my first language and that I spoke some Arabic, too, hoping for a competitive edge. Being a paralegal wasn't my ideal job—I didn't even really know what it entailed—but it seemed like the kind of thing a sensible person might do. Mostly, I thought that a change of scenery could save me from my increasingly reckless behavior. Moving to Paris wasn't a bucket list item: it was my escape plan.

A few nights before I left the city for good, I found myself at my third party of the evening, where investment bankers in upturned collars sat hunched over caterpillar-thick lines of cocaine, sweating as they talked animatedly about their stock portfolios, summer rentals in Montauk, and on and on. It was 5:00 A.M., and this wasn't my scene. I wanted to go home.

Standing alone on the sidewalk, bathed in the blue smoke of my cigarette, I watched the night sky begin to lighten around me. Manhattan was asleep in that fleeting hour of quiet after the garbage trucks finished their rounds and before the coffee shops opened. I'd been waiting for a taxi for ten minutes when a young man I recognized from the party strolled over, asking to bum a smoke. It was my last one but I handed it over. He lit the cigarette, cupping his hand, big as a baseball mitt, around the end. He smiled as he exhaled, the two of us shifting feet as we glanced shyly at each other, then stared down the empty street.

"Want to share?" he asked. A lone taxi was coming our way and the question seemed innocuous enough, so I said sure, and we climbed in. It was only after I'd given the driver my address that it occurred to me that the young man had asked me to split a ride without knowing where I was going.

I knew better than to get in cars with strange men. My father, who lived in the East Village in the eighties when the city was infested with crime, would have strongly disapproved. But there was something about the young man that felt safe and intriguing. His hair, shaggy and sun-streaked, flopped over intelligent blue eyes. Lean of build, square of jaw, and dimpled of cheek, he was strikingly handsome, but had terrible posture, carrying himself with a humility that suggested he was unaware of his looks.

"You might be the tallest person I've ever met," I said, studying him out of the corner of my eye. A towering six feet, six inches, he sat with his knees scrunched against the back of the driver's seat.

"So I've heard," he replied. He spoke softly and had a gentleness to him, despite his stature.

"It's nice to meet you. I'm—"

"We talked earlier, remember?"

I shrugged, then flashed him an apologetic smile. "It's been a long night."

"You don't remember when you tried to show me the inside of your eyelid? Or when you recited 'Mary Had a Little Lamb' in Latin?" he teased. "How about when you sprinkled pencil shavings on your head and kept saying *cascarones!* in a scary way? You don't remember any of that?"

"Ha. Ha. Very funny," I said, playfully punching his arm. It was then that I realized we were flirting.

He reached over to shake my hand. "I'm Will."

We talked the entire ride downtown, the chemistry between us intensifying with each city block. When we reached my apartment building, we both got out of the taxi and stood on the sidewalk: me considering if I should invite him upstairs, him too polite to ask. I had never gone to bed with a stranger before—despite some of the eyebrow-raising decisions I'd made, I had always been a bit of a romantic and a serial monogamist—but I was tempted. I mulled it over for a moment. "Hungry?" Will asked.

"Famished," I replied; relieved, I steered him away from the entrance to my building. We walked along Canal Street, past the shuttered hair-weave emporiums, roasted ducks hanging in deli windows, and sidewalk fruit vendors setting up their cardboard stands. We stepped into the neighborhood coffee joint, the first customers of the day.

Over bagels and coffee, Will began telling me about how he'd recently moved from China, where he'd worked for a sports organization, spearheading athletic outreach programs for local youth. I was impressed to learn he spoke Mandarin. At the moment, he was house-sitting for his godparents, and taking a couple of weeks to figure out his next steps. He was earnest and goofy, in a nerdy, dad-joke way. But beneath Will's easygoing façade, I sensed that he was a bit lost, and more than a little vulnerable. Two hours later

we were still there, still talking. *I really like you,* I remember thinking as we stood up to leave. My second thought was: *I wish I
weren't moving to a different continent.*

After breakfast, Will and I walked back to my building and up
the flight of stairs to my room. We spent all day in bed, napping
and chatting and joking around. I was used to guys who were ag-
gressively forward, armed with an arsenal of slick pickup lines,
but Will seemed content just to lie there side by side. When, after
several hours he still hadn't attempted to kiss me, I rolled over to
face him and made the first move. In the end, we did have that one-
night stand—and then a two- and three-night one. With him, it
was different; I left the lights on. I didn't feel the need to hide anything. He was the kind of guy who makes you look more generously on the parts of yourself that fill you with self-loathing. He
was the kind of guy who, if the circumstances had been different,
I would have taken my time getting to know.

On my last morning in New York, lemon-colored light filtered
in through the kitchen as I made coffee, the angry bleats of taxis
and sighs of buses down below faintly audible. I tiptoed into the
bedroom, collecting a few last articles of clothing and shoving
them into my suitcase. As I zipped it closed, I looked over at Will's
lanky figure tangled in sheets, his face angelic with sleep. He
looked so peaceful lying there that I didn't want to wake him. A
childhood spent on the move had made me weary of goodbyes. On
my way out, I left a note on his shoes saying, *Thanks for the unexpected fun. Inshallah, our paths will cross again someday.*

2

MÉTRO, BOULOT, DODO

IF MANHATTAN IS where people move to jump-start careers, Paris is where they go to live out the fantasy of a different life, and that was exactly what I intended to do. Stepping out of the *métro* and onto the streets of Le Marais, I walked with my bulky red suitcase clunking behind me, pausing every few feet to ogle the sidewalk cafés, boulangeries, and vine-covered façades of my new neighborhood. Through a friend of a friend, I had been lucky enough to find a furnished studio to rent in an eighteenth-century building on rue Dupetit-Thouars. I rode the rickety, wrought iron freight elevator up to the third floor. As I unlocked the front door, the contrast between Canal Street and my new place made me want to dance on the doormat with joy. *Light! Quiet! Privacy! Hardwood floors! An oversize pink bathtub shaped like a clamshell!* The apartment couldn't have been bigger than four hundred square feet but to me it seemed palatial, and it was all mine.

I spent the weekend getting settled in, unpacking, opening a bank account, buying new sheets, and scouring the kitchen. On

Monday morning I took the *métro* to the law firm, which was located in an elegant townhouse adjacent to the Parc Monceau in the eighth arrondissement. A fleet of paralegals greeted me in the lobby, their heels clicking along the polished marble floors as they gave me a tour. I'd held all kinds of odd jobs from the time I was a teenager—dog walker, babysitter, personal assistant, double bass teacher, restaurant hostess—but it was my first time working in a corporate environment. The office had twenty-foot ceilings with elaborate crown moldings, gold-framed paintings, and a grand twisting staircase. The lawyers sat at their wooden desks, cigarettes in one hand, espressos in the other, which struck me as very French and very chic. At noon, a group of us went to a café around the corner for a languorous lunch and ordered steaks and two bottles of wine, expensed to the firm. When I returned, I was given a BlackBerry for work use and shown the supply closet. Equipped with a stack of bright yellow legal pads and sophisticated pens, I sat at my desk, feeling very grown-up as I leaned back in my chair and lit a cigarette, glancing around my new surroundings with glee.

Rather than taking the subway I decided to walk home after my first day of work. At dusk, the narrow, crooked alleys of Le Marais took on a medieval cast. The streetlamps sputtered to life, and as I wandered, I fantasized about the person I could now become. Gone were the friends who were not really my friends at all—just people with an appetite for mischief and late nights. Even the itch seemed to have subsided. With an ocean lying between me and all that, I imagined myself spending quiet, solitary weekends exploring the city, picnicking in the Tuileries Garden and reading a good book at a little café I'd discovered around the corner. I would get a bicycle with a basket that I would fill with groceries each Sunday at the outdoor market on Place de la République. I would start wearing red lipstick and heels like the other paralegals. I would learn to cook my aunt Fatima's famous couscous and host dinner parties in my new home. Determined to spend less time talking about the things I wanted to do and more time actually doing them, I would sign up for one of the fiction workshops at Shakespeare and Company, the famous bookstore on the banks of the Seine. Maybe I'd even get a dog, a chubby King Charles spaniel that I would name Chopin.

But I didn't have free time, and the few Sundays I made it to the market, the produce sat in my fridge until it mossed over with mold. Instead, I was thrust into a life that the French describe as *"métro, boulot, dodo"* (subway, work, sleep). By the end of my first week of work, it was clear to me that I was not cut out for a career in law. I preferred creative writing to spreadsheets, Birkenstocks to high heels. The firm specialized in international arbitration, which had sounded interesting to me at first, but whenever I tried to read the briefs that came across my desk, I found the legal jargon inscrutable, the content mind-numbingly tedious. The majority of my days were spent in the office basement, proofreading, printing, and collating thousands of documents into neatly organized binders so that the lawyers could help soulless corporations get richer. Expected to be on call 24/7, I slept with my work phone on my pillow and set alarms for the middle of the night so that I could check for urgent emails. Often, I didn't get to leave the office at all; the paralegals pulled so many all-nighters that we began to keep score. On top of all this, I had a creepy boss who stashed catalogs of women's shoes in his desk drawer and, when he thought I wasn't looking, snapped photographs of my feet with his phone. After clocking yet another ninety-hour week, my way of letting loose was grabbing a *pain au chocolat* on the run and going out dancing. At the end of a late night out, I'd drag whomever I was with to an old jazz club called Aux Trois Mailletz, where we'd sing off-key at the piano and drink wine until our lips were purple.

My life in Paris was not the fantasy I'd imagined, but I began to concoct a different version. My correspondence with Will started unexpectedly, the short, hey-what's-up-how's-it-going text messages turning into long, quippy email exchanges followed by fat envelopes stuffed with handwritten letters and thoughtfully annotated *New Yorker* stories. Will sent me a postcard from a cabin in the White Mountains of New Hampshire where he'd gone away with friends for a weekend: *No electricity, a wood-burning stove from the early 1900s, and no sounds but owls, crackling fire and the wind,* he wrote. *It made me want to travel the back roads of the US. Want to take a road trip?* The idea of us driving together across the country made my heart do a little two-step.

At the bottom of our letters we always signed off the same way—*no need to write back in equal word count*—but our exchanges grew deeper and more frequent as the weeks and months passed. I read each of his letters over and over as if they were encrypted maps that offered secret clues and insights into the person holding the pen. I told Will about my wayward path since graduation and my new life abroad: *I spent my first 36 hours in Paris in total solitude with my laptop and cell phone turned off. I walked all over the city, until the heel on my shoe broke and I had to take a taxi home.* Despite my best attempts at a more ascetic life, I had picked up a new cast of friends—Lahora, a widowed yogi; Zack, an old college classmate who was training to be a mime; Badr, a young Moroccan businessman who loved to go out dancing; and David, an elderly expat who dressed like an international playboy and threw extravagant parties. *You can't force solitude onto a soul that needs to fly,* Will replied. At such a line, how could I help but swoon?

I told Will about my dream of becoming a journalist and shared with him an essay about the Arab-Israeli conflict that I'd been laboring over for months. What a coincidence, he responded; he, too, had journalistic ambitions. He had recently taken a job as a research assistant to a professor and was hoping to find work as an editor, and he sent me thoughtful notes on how I might revise my draft. Despite our time together during my final week in New York, these small moments of connection came as a surprise, for it was only through letter writing that we began to really know each other, our old-fashioned correspondence offering a safer, more honest alternative to the cat-and-mouse games of dating. Soon, I grew so smitten with my new pen pal that he was all I thought about, dreamed about, talked about, anymore. I hoped that the person off the page might be as wonderful as the one conjured from ink.

It was a late-autumn afternoon, a rare slow day at the office, and I was debating with Kamilla, the paralegal with whom I shared a desk, about whether I should invite Will to visit me in Paris. I wasn't sure if the romantic subtext of our letters was in my head, but I worried that if I didn't take the initiative soon, our correspondence would peter out. Over the next hour, I composed several different drafts of an email to Will, trying to strike the right tone, somewhere between earnest enthusiasm and detached cool. "*Allez ma chérie, courage,* at this rate you're going to be here all night," Kamilla said, pecking me on the cheek before heading out.

By the time I settled on a final version, it was dark out, the office nearly empty. I counted to ten, feeling more than a little immature as I dared myself to hit Send. When I finally worked up the guts to do it, I felt a thrill—only to have that quickly eclipsed by the anxiety of waiting for him to respond. Time seemed to trickle by. I smoked half a pack of Gauloises, I surfed the Web, I reorganized my desk. At nine, I finally took the *métro* home. I checked my email. Still nothing. I fretted as I fixed myself a dinner of Nutella-slathered toast. Had I overstepped or misread the vibe? Before bed, I would take a bath and then, if there was still no response, I would purge him from my head.

At midnight, I checked one last time. A message had arrived in my in-box. I opened it and discovered a forwarded flight confirmation. Destination: Paris, France.

.   .   .

Will arrived a little less than a month later, just in time for Thanksgiving. I spent the weekend before in a frenzy of preparations. I scrubbed the bathtub until it shone, swept the floors clear of dust motes, and hauled my sheets to the laundromat. I went to the Marché des Enfants Rouges and picked out a loaf of bread and a smelly wheel of Camembert, grabbed a jar of cornichons, sheets of charcuterie, and a bouquet of dried lavender. On the way home I bought some wine and, at the last minute, ducked into the salon across the street for a much-needed trim. On the morning of Will's arrival, I rose at dawn and changed my outfit no fewer than six times before settling on my most flattering pair of jeans, a tight black turtleneck, and my good-luck gold hoops. By the time I set out for the airport, I was running almost an hour late.

A misty breeze swept across rue Dupetit-Thouars as the heels of my boots clicked hard and fast against the rain-slicked sidewalk. I was nearly at the *métro* when I heard my phone ping. It was a text from Will saying his flight had landed early and that he'd taken a taxi straight to my address; someone had let him into the building and he was waiting outside my apartment door. Hotfooting it back to my building, I took the steps two at a time, pausing when I reached the second-floor landing to compose myself. My heart was beating like a jacked-up metronome, my forehead was clammy, my breathing ragged. I had noticed in recent weeks that I seemed to get winded more easily. I made a mental note to look into a gym membership. Brushing my hair out of my face, I took a deep inhale and turned the corner.

"Hey, hey!" Will called out when he caught sight of me, his posture straightening and his face crinkling into a big, toothy grin. We hesitated for a moment before hugging, both of us suddenly too timid to attempt a kiss, even on the cheek. Wrapped in the arms of a man who was not quite a stranger but not much more than that, I felt, for the first time in months, that I was standing on steady ground.

"*Bienvenue,*" I said when we disentangled, and I ushered him inside. My studio was tiny and other than the kitchen and the bathroom, it was just one all-purpose room. "This is the bedroom," I said, gesturing to the loft bed. "This is the living room," I said, pointing to the bright red couch. "This is the dining room," I said, showing him the old steamer trunk that also functioned as coffee table, desk, and cupboard. It was the first place I had ever lived alone and, although it was a bit spartan and I still hadn't found time to buy curtains, I was proud of it. "And voilà!" I said, completing the tour as I threw open the big bay windows to reveal a small terrace.

"The best," Will confirmed.

The rest of the day is hazy, and it comes to me in snapshots: the nervous chitchat in the living room as we drank coffee, the dozen individually wrapped gifts Will laid out on the trunk, the meandering stroll along the Seine, where we laughed at the sight of American study abroad students sporting berets and speaking terrible French. "Don't even *think* about kissing me here," I warned, as we crossed the Pont des Arts, where lovers affixed padlocks to the bridge's grillwork. It was only later that night, after a bottle of red wine had loosened our nerves, that he did.

Will followed me up the ladder to the loft bed, a cheap, rickety affair made up of four wooden posts and a flimsy plywood platform that the previous tenant had assembled, dubiously. As we lay side by side, it felt different from those three nights we shared back in New York. A tender awkwardness filled the air as we undressed. Moonlight poured in through the window, turning the scars on my legs a silvery hue. Beneath us, the bedposts swayed.

"Damn you, IKEA," I said.

"What if the bed collapses?" Will was genuinely concerned.

"Imagine my dad reading the newspaper headlines tomorrow: NAKED AMERICAN COUPLE FOUND DEAD IN PILE OF IKEA DEBRIS."

Will jumped down the ladder—"One sec, I need to perform an

evaluation." He checked that the bolts were screwed in properly, wiggling and shaking the frame as I laughed. "A seismic evaluation!"

At the end of his two-week visit, Will returned to New York, but only to pack up his things and quit his job. *He is moving to Paris to be with me*—I wrote in my journal again and again until it began to feel real. As I sat on the *métro* on my way to work, a stupid smile stretched across my face. *Joy is a terrifying emotion, don't trust it,* I added to the page. For under the joy, a storm was gaining speed, a roiling sense of foreboding, some wet, starless savagery unfolding beneath my skin.

3

EGGSHELLS

I HADN'T BEEN single for longer than a month or two since the age of seventeen. I wasn't proud of this, and I didn't think it was healthy, but that was how it had been. For the bulk of my time in college, I was in a serious relationship with a brilliant British-Chinese comparative literature major. He was my first real boyfriend and he took me to fancy dinners in the city and on vacation to Waikiki Beach, but as the semesters passed I grew restless, wishing I'd had more experience prior to meeting him. The summer before senior year, that relationship ended when I had a fiery fling with a young Ethiopian filmmaker. After that, it was a Bostonian I met while doing research over winter break in Cairo; he had a flair for grand-scale pranks and activism and had just been arrested for dropping a thirty-foot Palestinian flag down the side of one of the pyramids. A week later, as we drank bootleg whiskey at a bar overlooking the Red Sea, he dialed up his parents. "Meet the girl I'm gonna marry," he announced, passing the phone to me before I could protest. I broke up with him not long after. Around graduation I started seeing the Mexican-Texan aspiring screen-writer. We dated for two disastrous months in New York while I interned and he waited tables at a trendy downtown hotel. He got mean when he was drunk, and he was drunk most of the time.

There was nothing casual about these relationships. When I was in them, I was fully in them, consumed by the idea of a life together. But even during the most intense periods, I was aware of an exit sign glowing faintly in the distance—and the truth was, I was always on the verge of running for it. I was in love with the idea of being in love. Another way to say it is that I was young: too impulsive and reckless with the emotions of others, too self-involved and focused on figuring out what came next for me to dwell on broken promises.

With Will, it was different. He was unlike any man I'd been with before. He possessed a bizarre combination of traits—part jock, part intellectual, part class clown—and could dunk a basket-ball just as effortlessly as he could recite verses of W. B. Yeats's poems. I was taken aback by his thoughtfulness, by the way he was always intent on making everyone in a room feel at ease. Five years my senior, he had a quiet, unassuming wisdom and playful-ness of spirit that made him seem both far older and younger than his age. The moment Will returned to the doorstep of my Paris apartment, this time with an oversize duffel bag stuffed with all of his possessions, the exit sign disappeared from view. I was all in.

Will unpacked and folded his clothes into neat little stacks on the bookshelf I'd emptied to make room for his belongings. Rooting around in his duffel, he pulled out a portable speaker and asked if he could play some music. Nineties hip-hop, with Warren G on heavy rotation, boomed throughout the apartment. Laughter bub-bled up inside of me as he rapped along to the lyrics and danced across the hardwood floor. He took my hand and spun me around the kitchen, nearly knocking over a frying pan.

"You're distracting me," I said, swatting him away with a dish towel.

I was making shepherd's pie for lunch, wanting to impress Will with my culinary skills. With great concentration, I chopped carrots, sautéed shallots, browned meat, and mashed potatoes. Aside from scrambled eggs, the occasional bowl of pasta, and my go-to dinner of Nutella toast, it was the first dish from scratch I'd ever attempted, and I'd called my mom earlier that morning for the recipe. The kitchen was the size of a small utility closet, and without windows or a fan for ventilation, it was sweltering. I wiped my forehead with the dish towel and it beaded again as I layered all of the ingredients into a casserole dish and sprinkled a little cheese on top before putting the whole mess into the oven. Soon, the apartment smelled of butter and fresh herbs; it smelled for the first time like a real home.

In the other room, Will was setting the table on the steamer trunk. I joined him, cracking open the windows to let in a little air. It had started snowing outside, and a few lazy flakes drifted into the apartment. Will joined me at the window and hooked his arms around my waist, pulling me to him. "Tomorrow, I'll start looking for work," he said, burying his face into my hair. "I should also find a language school, somewhere I can take lessons, at least until I learn enough French to say 'I'll have three baguettes and an Orangina, please.'"

The muscles of Will's torso were taut and warm against my shoulder blades. I closed my eyes, softening into him, and tried to remember when I'd last felt this happy. Couldn't. "Stay right there," Will said, backing away. From the bookshelf, he grabbed his camera and snapped a photograph of me in front of the window, silhouetted against the winter sky. When he showed me the photograph, I was alarmed by my appearance. My skin looked so pale it was nearly translucent. My eyelids were a robin's-egg blue, as if all of the veins had floated to the surface. Even my lips looked drained of life force.

"The color of pearls," Will said generously, planting a kiss on them.

Two weeks later, Will turned twenty-seven years old. To celebrate his recent move and his birthday I took a few days off work and surprised him with an envelope containing two train tickets to Amsterdam. It was January 2011 and as we stepped out of the station our breath plumed in the bright morning air. We were hoping to explore the city by foot. On the itinerary: a visit to the Anne Frank House, a pit stop at the market to sample pickled herring, and a boat tour through the canals. But we didn't get far. Every block or so, I halted to a stop, a deep cough racking my body, leaving me light-headed and dizzy, my temples throbbing like tuning forks.

I felt so run-down that we ended up spending most of the weekend at our seedy, two-star hotel in the red-light district. The hotel's sheets were pocked with burn marks, a grimy window overlooked a canal, and the clackety-bang of a misfiring radiator echoed down the dreary halls. But the thing about being in love is that you can be anywhere and it feels like an adventure. In fact, when we'd first arrived, I'd turned to him and said excitedly, "This is my favorite hotel ever!"

Though I wasn't feeling well, I was determined that our first trip together be a memorable one. This is how, on the afternoon of Will's birthday, I found myself in a basement coffee shop, buying a tin of psychedelic mushrooms from a gangly white boy with dreadlocks. "Come on, don't be a square," I said to Will, who had never tried them before and seemed apprehensive. "Okay fine," he eventually agreed. "If the Mayans were on point, this is the last year for humankind. Let's do it right." We walked a few blocks to an Ethiopian restaurant for dinner, and when the waiter wasn't looking, I sprinkled a handful of the shrooms over a thick stew of spiced lentils. "You're a nut, you know that?" Will laughed, shaking his head at me as he skeptically scooped up the laced lentils with a piece of *injera*.

The fog hung low over the city as we headed back to the hotel after dinner. Trudging through the slushy streets and over icy bridges, we dodged cyclists who rang their bells as they flew past. As we wandered the red-light district, silhouettes glowed behind curtained windows. A traffic light turned orange, red, green, then burst into a rainbow. I could see our hotel from where we stood, its neon sign flickering like an ember. We quickened our pace, trying to reach our room before the drugs hit full force. By the time we got inside, the pores of my skin had turned into tiny torches emitting flames. I tore off all of my clothes and sprawled onto the mattress, attempting to cool off. Meanwhile, Will began building a fort from sheets and pillows, forming a tent over the bed. "Get in here, it's very *gezellig*," I said, patting the empty space next to me. *Gezellig*, the untranslatable Dutch expression, which roughly means "cozy," had become our new favorite word. Will slid under the canopy of sheets and lay down beside me.

"Jesus, you're burning up," he said, placing a palm onto my forehead.

In the moment, I thought it just meant the drugs were working, and working well. But over the next few hours, my fever crept up and up until my body felt like it might combust. I started shivering. Rivulets of sweat pooled in the hollows of my collarbones, and I remember feeling fragile for the first time in my life. "It's like I'm made of eggshells," I told him again and again. "Let's stay here forever, okay?"

Will grew concerned and suggested we go to the emergency room. "Let me take care of you," he said.

"*Non merci,* I am tough," I said, showing him my bicep.

"We can take a taxi straight there and we'll be back before you know it."

I refused, shaking my head no until he gave up. I didn't want to be one of those blundering tourists who traveled to Amsterdam, did a bunch of shrooms, and ended up in the hospital.

The next afternoon, we boarded a train back to Paris. The fever and the hallucinations had dissipated, but that feeling of fragility remained. With each passing day, I felt weaker, less vibrant. It was as if someone were taking an eraser to my core. The silhouette of my old self was still perceptible, but my insides were muting into a ghostly palimpsest.

4

SPACE TRAVELING

AND GAINING MOMENTUM

BACK IN PARIS, I went to see a doctor for the usual reason twenty-two-year-old girls do: birth control. The clinic was a dingy labyrinth of paint-chipped walls, crowded waiting rooms, and flickering overhead bulbs. The other patients, most of whom appeared to be immigrants, also of North African descent, spoke among themselves in a mix of Arabic and French as they wrangled squirmy toddlers or flipped through magazines. As I looked around, I felt a pang of homesickness. The transition from my lollipop-pocketed pediatrician who had known me most of my life to this cold, run-down clinic was a jarring reminder that I was now on my own. I wasn't a kid anymore, but I felt ill-equipped for the fluorescent, bureaucratic world of adulthood.

Eventually, my name was called. A phlebotomist cuffed the sleeve of my blouse and examined my arm for a usable vein. For as long as I could remember, I had been terrified of needles. Turning my face away, I glued my gaze to the ground and held my breath as the syringe pierced skin. Out of the corner of my eye, I saw the spurt of crimson. No biggie, I told myself. I exhaled as the tube filled. Almost done.

An hour or so later, I was ushered into the doctor's office, where a mustachioed man in a lab coat sat on the other side of a large wooden desk. I took a seat. "What brings you here today?" he asked me in French.

"I'd like to go on the pill," I said.

"That shouldn't be a problem." He glanced down at a piece of paper, reviewing the results of my blood test, and paused, his brow furrowing slightly. "Before we discuss the different options, I'm wondering if you've been feeling tired?"

I nodded vigorously.

"Your blood work shows you're anemic—that your red blood cell count is low." I must have looked troubled. "Don't worry," he added, "anemia is quite common in young women. Do you have a heavy menstrual period?"

I shrugged, unsure of what "heavy" constituted. "I guess." After a decade of cramps, any menstruation was too much menstruation in my book.

"That might be it, then," the doctor said. "I'll prescribe you the birth control and a daily iron supplement. That should give you more energy soon."

On the *métro* ride home, I counted down the stops to rue Dupetit-Thouars, still giddy at the novelty of coming home to a man and an apartment that were mine. Bursting through the door, cheeks ruddy from the cold, I gave Will a hug, then as I uncorked a bottle of wine, I told him about the anemia and the iron supplements. "That's why I've been feeling so freaking *fatiguée*." I felt hopeful and smiled at him. "How was your day?"

"Mila scraped her elbow on the merry-go-round at Champ de Mars and cried, but I was able to calm her down and everything was fine. So I would say it was a pretty *bonne journée*." Will was

taking French classes and had started working as a manny—
a male nanny—something I was expressly forbidden from calling
him, but did anyway, as often as possible. Every afternoon, while I
was at the law firm, he picked up four-year-old Mila from pre-
school and took her to various extracurriculars. She had chubby
cheeks and a frizzy cloud of brown curls. Her favorite activity was
sitting on Will's shoulders, where she had an aerial view of the
street action, while munching on a croissant and shouting to anyone who would listen, "I'm the tallest girl in all of Paris!" As Will
recounted their latest adventure, I picked flaky pastry crumbs out
of his hair.

The manny gig was temporary, just until Will found his footing
in Paris, and though he was hardly putting his diploma to good
use, he didn't seem to mind. It was steady, under-the-table cash
that didn't require him to have a work visa, and there were worse
ways to spend your afternoons than discovering a foreign city with
a four-year-old guide. I, on the other hand, was less optimistic
about my job. I had been finding it difficult to get through the
workday. The itch had lessened since I'd moved to Paris, but the
exhaustion was so all-consuming that I was drinking up to eight
espressos a day. I started to worry that my deep weariness might be
something else. *Maybe I just can't cut it in the real world,* I'd written in my journal. But the doctor at the clinic had offered an alternative explanation: anemia, which meant my fatigue was *of me,*
not *about me,* a distinction for which I was grateful.

It grew late, and the wine bottle now sat empty on the trunk. I
swayed to my feet and declared we were long overdue for our resolutions, which we'd planned to make on New Year's Eve a few
weeks earlier. I loved the annual ritual of drafting resolutions: I
was always filling journals with to-do lists and dreams. The sem-
blance of a plan, no matter how tenuous, balanced out the uncertainty and confusion I felt about the future. Though Will wasn't
much of a planner, he humored me. Come spring, he said, he
would apply to graduate school, maybe at Sciences Po, the Paris

Institute of Political Studies. I vowed to find a new job, one that didn't leave me devoid of energy at the end of each day, something other than making photocopies or hiding my feet from my boss.

Over the next two months, I tried to make good on my resolution: I spruced up my résumé, sent out job applications, and reached out to former professors and mentors for advice. But mostly, I found myself back in the clinic's dreary waiting room, where I returned half a dozen times to be treated for various colds, bouts of bronchitis, and urinary tract infections. Each time, I was assigned to a different doctor. Each time, I gave my medical history anew, the list of recent ailments growing longer by the visit. I was taking the iron supplements as instructed, but instead of feeling revitalized, I felt more and more depleted. The rotating cast of doctors at the clinic made me wonder who was keeping track of all the details—who, if anyone, had my back.

One afternoon, as I was getting yet another "routine" blood test, I felt tears fill my eyes. "What's wrong?" the phlebotomist asked.

I wasn't sure anymore.

The thing about being tired all day, every day, for many months is that you don't notice yourself getting sicker. By the time I got a referral to see a doctor at the American Hospital of Paris, I had grown so weak that it was a struggle to climb up and down the ladder of the loft bed. On an unseasonably warm Friday afternoon in late March I left home for the appointment. What should have been a thirty-minute *métro* ride took hours, and I ended up in a neighborhood of Paris I didn't recognize. I wandered in circles, searching for the hospital only to realize I had gotten off at the wrong stop. As I waited for a bus that would take me to Neuilly-sur-Seine, a western suburb of Paris where the hospital was located, I felt dazed. All around me, grand homes and expensive cars shimmered in the sun. Birds fluttered through the heart-shaped leaves of a linden tree. A mother walked hand in hand with her two blond children down the shady side of the street. My head began to spin. Starbursts dotted my vision and suddenly the houses, the cars, the birds, the mother dwindled to flecks of gold against pitch black. One minute I was standing; the next, I'd fallen sideways, my head slamming the sidewalk.

"*Ça va,* mademoiselle?" an elderly lady asked when I came to, her papery lips pinched in concern.

"*Non,*" I answered, as I began to cry again. I couldn't reach Will, who was with Mila at her weekly swimming lesson, and my parents were four thousand miles away. I was space traveling and gaining momentum, spinning farther and farther away from Earth. I had never felt so alone.

When I finally arrived at the hospital, it was dusk. A man who introduced himself as Dr. K took a quick look at me on the examining room table and decided to admit me to the hospital to run further tests. "*Vous n'avez vraiment pas bonne mine,*" he told me. (Translation: You look like crap.) An orderly pushed me upstairs in a wheelchair to a white room with a large window. The sun was setting and I watched as dark purple clouds rolled across the horizon, threatening rain. The last time I'd spent the night in a hospital had been when I was born.

The American Hospital of Paris looked unlike any stateside hospital I had ever seen. My room was luxurious, bigger than my studio, and the walls were whitewashed in sunlight. I looked forward to the breakfast trays that arrived at my bedside each morning unbidden, the aromas of a buttery croissant and a café au lait stirring me from sleep. With breakfast came a daily dose of prednisone, a garden-variety steroid, prescribed to me for reasons that remained unclear, but within seventy-two hours, it had me feeling chipper enough to walk downstairs to the hospital courtyard, where I spent the afternoons writing in my journal, bumming cigarettes off the other cotton-robe-clad patients, and gazing, glassy-eyed, out onto the flower beds. In the evenings, after tucking Mila into bed, Will joined me at the hospital. He brought Scrabble, and we stayed up late talking and playing game after game. A nurse had offered him a visitor's cot so he could stay over.

"Thank you for being here," I murmured groggily, as we fell asleep in our separate beds.

"It makes me the happiest person to be with you, it's been the happiest few months of my life," Will said, reaching for my hand. "There's no one quite like you. No one who urges me to live more than you do—who makes me want to be *me* more than you do. Your appetite for knowing more, and knowing yourself better, makes me want to be better. What we're building together is big. And soon you'll be out of here, and we can get back to our life."

During my weeklong stay in the hospital, the doctors ran every test they could conceive of, from HIV to lupus to cat scratch fever. All negative. I answered countless questions: Nope, no prior surgeries or hospitalizations; no medical conditions; one grandfather died of prostate cancer, the other one from a heart attack, but otherwise no known family history of illness; if you count dancing in nightclubs, then yes, I exercise regularly. When Dr. K looked at my red blood cells under a microscope, he found that they were enlarged and mentioned something about my possibly needing a bone marrow biopsy. "How much alcohol do you drink?" he asked me one afternoon, standing over my bed. "Too much," I piped back. "I did recently graduate from college." I watched him jot down notes on a pad of paper as he walked out of the room. In the end, he decided that a biopsy was unnecessary for someone my age. I trusted him. After all, youth and health are supposed to go hand in hand.

"You need rest," Dr. K concluded. "I'm still puzzled by your red blood cells, but I don't see any reason for alarm. I'm going on vacation but let's follow up when I get back in a couple of weeks and see how you feel." With that, he discharged me with a diagnosis of something called "burnout syndrome" and granted me a one-month medical leave from work.

On the *métro* ride home from the hospital, I wrote in my journal:

Important Medical Details to Remember:

1) Dr. K wears Prada glasses.
2) Will and I almost got caught having sex in the bathroom of my hospital room by a nurse.
3) You can order crème brûlée and champagne directly to your room from the hospital cafeteria.
4) I'm pretty sure this place is a country club disguised as a hospital.
5) WTF is "burnout syndrome"?

Admittedly, I was psyched about the monthlong leave from my job, but the rest wasn't fully adding up. Without the daily dose of prednisone, my energy was already waning. Slumped against the cold plastic *métro* seat, fighting to stay awake, it dawned on me that Dr. K might have thought that hard work and heavy play were the only culprits here. I didn't feel he, or any of the other doctors I'd seen, were taking me seriously. But I can't say I was either. I didn't speak up. Instead, I dismissed the doubts ping-ponging inside my head. They were the ones with the medical degrees, not me.

A few days after returning home from the hospital I awoke to the good news that I had a job interview. I'd spent the last few weeks sending out inquiries to various newspapers and magazines with little success. Unlike other careers, where there were clear-cut paths to follow, corporate ladders to climb, or necessary degrees to obtain, the world of journalism was as mystifying to me as it was inaccessible. I had no idea how to get my foot in the door. "Just start writing and pitching stories to editors," someone had told me, but my day job didn't leave much time for that. Even if it had, I didn't know any editors and even if I did, I likely wouldn't have had the confidence to put myself out there. So instead I had written to my old journalism professor, who suggested I reach out to the *International Herald Tribune,* which was headquartered in Paris, about potential entry-level positions. To my surprise, they responded, saying they had an opening for a "stringer," a kind of low-level information gatherer who would help their more senior reporters cover the revolution that had just broken out in Tunisia— later known as the Arab Spring. They wanted me to come in for an interview right away.

The next day, I put on a black tailored dress I'd scored from a thrift store, tamed my tangled curls into a braid, applied an extra swipe of blush across my pallid cheeks, and set out for the interview. Huffing up the stairs of the *Tribune* office, I noted the familiar light-headedness returning, my breath just out of reach, but there were more important things to focus on that day. The sound of clacking keyboards filled the office, an open-floor plan crammed with filing cabinets and desks piled high with books, computer monitors, and dirty coffee mugs. Looking around at the cast of seasoned reporters sitting at their desks, I didn't allow myself any illusions. I knew my chances of getting the job were slim, but for the first time, I could see a path toward a profession that excited me. Suddenly I realized that, without meaning to, this was what I'd been preparing for. In school, I'd crammed my semesters full of language courses—Arabic, French, Spanish, Farsi—with the idea that one day I could live and work in far-flung locales with greater ease. I'd spent each of my summers studying and doing research abroad, which had allowed me to travel everywhere from Addis Ababa and Morocco's Atlas Mountains to the West Bank. As for Tunisia, it wasn't just a country that I knew and loved, it was the homeland: where my father was from, where all of my extended family still lived, and from where I proudly held a passport. All this came out in the interview, and the editors I met with seemed delighted. I was, too. I left thinking that I'd been working toward just that moment my entire adult life, then laughed at myself—all four years of it.

I never returned to the *Tribune* office. Within a week, I was back in the hospital. This time, I lay on a gurney in the emergency room, my eyes bleached blank with pain. Throbbing sores colonized the inside of my mouth. My complexion was blue-gray, like dead meat. Will squeezed my hand as the doctor on call said: "I don't want you to panic, but something's clearly going on. Your red blood cell count has dropped significantly." I stared at her, not knowing what any of this meant. "If it drops any lower you won't be allowed to board a plane." She placed a hand gently on my arm, and went on to say that she had a daughter about my age, and that if she were my mother she'd want me on the next flight home.

Arrangements were made for me to fly back to New York first thing the following morning. I also insisted on purchasing a return ticket to Paris for two weeks later. I needed to believe that this would be a round-trip journey. Will had offered to accompany me, but in my mind that didn't make sense—he had to take care of Mila, and I would be back soon. As I said goodbye to him at the airport, I told him not to worry. Then an elderly man in a navy-blue uniform carted me off in a wheelchair through Charles de Gaulle. My ears burned as he pushed me to the front of the security lines and onto the plane, past the swarm of families waiting to board and the business travelers holding fancy leather briefcases. I thought surely the emergency room doctor had been overreacting when she'd insisted I use a wheelchair. I remember worrying that someone was going to call me out at any moment for being a fraud. But those in the priority boarding line who looked at me, if they noticed me at all, did so with a discernible sense of pity.

The plane took off. Curled in the fetal position across two empty seats, I shivered under a thin blanket, unable to get warm. I'd always loved planes, the sense of smallness that comes with altitude, the earth growing smaller and smaller until it vanishes beneath the clouds, but this time I kept the window shade drawn. I was too tired to do anything—to watch movies or to eat the snacks that the concerned stewardess kept offering me. But tired as I was, my cheeks, swollen from the sores, made it difficult to sleep. The emergency room doctor had prescribed codeine for the flight home and I swallowed a couple of pills, hoping for some respite from the pain. Waves of nausea broke over my body as my mind began to row in and out of consciousness.

I dreamed that the plane was a flying penitentiary suspended over the Atlantic and that I was being punished for all the booze and cigarettes and bad shit I had pumped into my body in the last year. I dreamed I was at my five-year college reunion and that my friends stood with their backs to me, laughing and sipping cocktails on a lush, lime-green lawn, the dorms rising up in the distance, sizzling under an orange sun. I called out to them, but when they turned they looked right through me. This made sense in dream logic. *Maybe they don't recognize me,* I thought. I had aged since graduation—badly. Sitting in the same airport wheelchair, I was all bones in a bag of skin, with only a few long threads of silvery hair hanging from my nearly bald skull. My pupils were milky with cataracts, my mouth a toothless gaping hole. I called out again. *It's me,* I shouted, *Suleika.* But this time no one turned around at all.

When I opened my eyes next I felt the thud of the plane's wheels hitting the runway. I was home.

5

STATESIDE

I'VE BEEN CALLING my parents by their first names from the time I learned to speak, something that never struck any of us as odd until a perplexed schoolteacher pointed it out.

My mother, Anne, a petite woman with ice-blue eyes and the slim, sinewy musculature of a ballerina, hails from a bucolic Swiss village an hour outside of Geneva. She grew up in a stone house filled with old books, antiques, and a gramophone that was always playing classical music. The living room windows opened onto a town square overlooking a medieval castle and a sparkling lake where my mother spent her weekends swimming laps and sailing with the neighborhood boys. She was a *garçon manqué*, tomboyish, her hair cut short, her nose always buried in a novel. Her father, Luc, a physicist and an environmental activist, was strict, bordering on militant, but also ahead of his time. He refused to own a car because of the carbon emissions and forbade the use of plastic in the house. In the attic, he kept a woodworking shop where he would make hand-carved toys for Anne and her three siblings. Her mother, Mireille, a librarian, was uninterested in her husband's activism. She loved beautiful things, had an impressive collection of cashmere sweaters and a sprawling rose garden, and was known for her stupendous Swiss apple tarts. There was a right and a wrong way to behave, Mireille always said, and she subjected her children to rigorous etiquette lessons. By the time Anne was a teenager, she was bucking under the constraints of her parents' edicts and the cloistered atmosphere of the village.

After finishing art school in Lausanne, my mother won a grant to move to New York City, where she intended to become a famous painter. She rented a small railroad apartment on the corner of Fourth Street and Avenue A in the East Village. It was the height of the eighties, and the neighborhood was a grid of graffitied tenements and derelict, rubble-filled lots. The streets bristled with energy, and everywhere there were young writers and musicians radiating creativity and ambition. She had never been anywhere like it.

Hustle is our family's defining trait. My mother had the work ethic of a draft horse and never stopped moving from dawn until dusk. She scrounged together a living by working as a house painter and selling roses table to table at restaurants and cafés, enough to rent both the apartment and a studio that she shared with a couple of artists. She soon found a more lucrative enterprise to pay the bills and began running a small business out of her apartment. "International Language School, how may I help you?" she would answer the phone, pretending to be a secretary. The school, if it could be called that, consisted of my mother and her friends, a crew that came from all over Europe. She hired them to give French, Italian, German, and Spanish language lessons to businesspeople and wealthy uptown families. She would eventually save enough to put a small down payment on her apartment, which was selling for forty thousand dollars, what seemed like a fortune at the time.

Five years into Anne's time in New York, her wit and cropped
hair, aristocratic nose and elegant cheekbones, captured my father
Hédi's attention at a downtown jazz club. It was no hard feat for
Hédi to win her over. Tall and tawny, with a mop of black curls
and a charming gap between his two front teeth, he had just run
the New York City Marathon and was in the best shape of his life.
He lived a few blocks away, on Seventh Street between Avenues B
and C, so close that they were soon seeing each other all the time.
They bonded over their shared lingua franca, their nomadism, and
their love of cooking, cinema, and the arts. They had the same
bohemian values, spending what money they had on good wine,
theater tickets, and travel, but they squabbled often, both of them
too stubborn and independent for their own good. My mother's
priority was her painting, and she had no interest in being anyone's wife. My father was still debating whether to stay in the
United States or to return to his homeland to settle down and make
a life. Two years into their courtship, I was conceived in Hédi's
apartment on Tompkins Square Park. *An accident,* I imagined my
mother thinking, already mourning her freedom, as she peed over
a stick. (Later she would revise this sentiment: *A surprise,* she
would tell me.)

At forty, Hédi was almost a decade older than Anne. He taught
high school at the United Nations International School and free-
lanced as a translator of French and Arabic. He was overjoyed by
the pregnancy, but Anne had difficulty seeing herself as a mother,
and she was unconvinced about marriage. Most of her friends
back home in Switzerland had partners and children without ever
officially getting hitched. Marriage struck her as stifling and old-
fashioned. She insisted they didn't need a piece of paper to legiti-
mize their relationship. A few months later, she changed her mind,
but only so that my father could comfortably share the news of the
pregnancy with his mother. They proceeded with a civil ceremony.
A Polaroid from that day shows them standing on the steps of City
Hall in downtown Manhattan, beaming at each other in oversize

suits as they hold their version of a bouquet: two branches, still tufted with leaves, that had been snapped off a scraggly city tree.

I know all this because my mother and I are close—no topic off-limits, no major life event unexplored. With her thick accent, pixie cut, unshaven armpits, and paint-splattered overalls, she wasn't like any of the other mothers I knew. When I got my period at thirteen, she was the first person I told, and the next day she surprised me with the world's most awkward celebratory luncheon, making emotional toasts about my nascent womanhood as my father and brother squirmed uncomfortably in their seats. As a teenager, I'd once told her that I planned to save my virginity until marriage. "Don't be an idiot," my mother replied. "You need to know what you like before you commit to something for life."

We were constantly on the move in those early years—from the East Village to the Adirondacks, followed by stints in France, Switzerland, and Tunisia, but we always returned to the United States, where my father had secured a tenure-track teaching position at Skidmore, a small liberal arts college in Saratoga Springs, New York. Despite her initial hesitations, Anne loved being a mother, and after my brother was born, she decided to scale back her career to focus on raising us. She approached parenting with the same creativity and zest that infused her abstract paintings of insects, flowers, and honeycombs—all of which ended up looking more or less like vaginas. During the snowy upstate winters, she would strap on her cross-country skis and a backward baseball cap and glide to our bus stop a few blocks away to pick us up. She turned the attic of our house into a studio, where she held art classes and where we spent our afternoons sitting cross-legged on the wide-planked floors, playing with gouache and watercolor sets. She taught us about pointillism, showing us the masterpieces of Georges Seurat and giving us Q-tips dipped in paint to make our own dotted landscapes.

Each night before bed, she would read us fables and fairy tales in French. If we had been extra good, she would massage us with almond oil. "What should we garden today?" she would say, kneading our backs as if tilling rocky soil, making us squeal as she pinched the skin beneath our shoulder blades to "plant seeds." She had a delightfully dark sense of humor and was notorious for her pranks, which she sometimes took a little too far. Once, on April Fools' Day, her favorite holiday of the year, she emailed my brother and me with the "grim news" that our father had lost his job, so we'd have to drop out of college immediately and get full-time jobs. Then she forgot all about it and went to the movies, leaving us to fret for hours. It was this sense of mischief and audacity that made her company feel so freeing and magical; it made her accessible, not like one of those grown-ups who constantly reminded you of your immaturity. After I left home, after I graduated and moved to a different time zone, the phone became our umbilical cord. We spoke every day, often multiple times.

My relationship to Hédi was a different story. He was an enigma to me. He grew up under French colonial rule in Gabès, a town in southern Tunisia with an oasis on the Mediterranean coast. Neither of his parents knew how to read or write. His father, Mahmoud, worked in the mail room at the town hall. He was loving but stern, a firm believer in the adage *"qui aime bien, châtie bien"*—spare the rod, spoil the child. His mother, Sherifa, was gentle and selfless, with a Berber tattoo on her chin and long henna-dyed braids that she kept covered with a scarf. My father joked that whenever he came home from school, Sherifa was always giving birth to a new baby. The family lived hand to mouth, and only seven of her thirteen children survived those postwar years of scarcity and disease. My father, the second eldest, wasn't the most studious of the bunch, but he was the most resourceful and determined to succeed. After graduating from the University of Tunis, he eventually made his way to London, then Paris, to further his studies, before immigrating to the United States, where he earned his doctorate in French literature.

I worshipped my professor-father with his dapper white linen suits and fedoras, head-turning looks, and dizzying memory for languages, but I was a little scared of him, too. He was a bon vivant, generous and brimming with charisma, but like his own father, he was quick to anger, his temper always threatening to boil over. He raised my younger brother, Adam, and me the same way he had been raised, a tough, compliments-make-you-soft school of parenting. He had no patience for childish antics. "Interesting people don't talk about gossip or idle events, they talk about *ideas,*" he would say to me whenever I was being too chatty or was otherwise getting on his nerves.

It was only during high school, once I had gotten serious about my studies, that my dad and I found some common ground. I loved sitting in the armchair in his office, reading his books. He had a floor-to-ceiling library filled with hundreds of volumes of classics, poetry, novels, and literary theory. Whenever I couldn't understand a word, I looked it up in one of the dictionaries on the bottom shelf, keeping a vocabulary list in the back of my journal. Under his guidance, I began to read in French, discovering the works of Baudelaire, Flaubert, Camus, Sartre, and Fanon. Although I had spoken some Arabic during the time we'd spent living in Tunisia when I was a kid, I had since forgotten it almost entirely, and became determined to relearn my father's native tongue. In college, inspired by his own academic interests, I'd majored in Near Eastern Studies with a double minor in French and Gender Studies. I'd sent my father every single paper I wrote and he labored over them for hours with a red pen, sending me revisions and suggestions for further reading. For my senior thesis, I'd traveled to Tunisia to gather the oral histories of older women, including my grandmother, and I interviewed them about the Code of Personal Status, a series of progressive postcolonial laws aimed at establishing equality between women and men. "*Je suis fier de toi,*" my father told me when I managed to graduate with highest honors and a handful of thesis prizes. It was a rare vocal display of parental pride.

As a graduation gift, my parents gave me a fire-engine-red suitcase, a big, boxy affair with smooth-gliding swivel wheels, bought
from the sale rack at T.J. Maxx. It came in handy later that summer when I got the Paris job. I remembered how optimistic my
parents seemed as they bade me bon voyage. *"Ton premier boulot!
Ça va être super!"* they said when they dropped me off at the airport. They insisted on taking a last, curbside photograph of me
with the suitcase, and I rolled heavily kohl-rimmed eyes to the sky,
flashing them a half-assed smile before sprinting into the terminal.
I was so preoccupied by what lay ahead that I almost forgot to turn
and give them a final wave goodbye. Little did any of us know that
I would be back seven months later. This time no one would be
taking pictures or chatting about my future plans.

An airport attendant helped me collect my suitcase and then
parked my wheelchair in the arrivals hall at John F. Kennedy International Airport. "Miss, you sure it's okay to leave you here?"

I nodded. My father was late to pick me up, as usual. Punctual-
ity had never been our family's strong suit.

As I waited, the revolving doors spat out one weary traveler
after another. Nearly an hour later, I spotted my father in his black
fedora, tilted to one side of his extremely bald head, and saw him
amble through the crowd. His eyes, dark and thick-lashed like a
dairy cow's, scanned the room, searching for someone who resembled his daughter. "Hédi," I shouted, flapping my arms in the air,
"Hédi, over here!"

I watched as the shock registered on my father's face, his features softening as he took in my swollen cheeks, my bluish lips,
and the sweatshirt that hung off my emaciated torso. He stooped
down to give me a kiss on the cheek. *"Salut, ma belle. Désolé,* I got
turned around on the freeway," he said. Pushing my wheelchair
with one hand and pulling the red suitcase with the other, he rolled
me toward the parking lot where the old family minivan was wait-

ing. I climbed into the backseat and lay down, too drained to say
much of anything during the three-and-a-half-hour drive to Saratoga Springs.

It's a funny thing, coming home. Everything smells the same, looks
the same, feels the same, but you are different; the contrast between who you were when you left and who you are now is heightened against the backdrop of old haunts. When we pulled up to
the house, where my family had lived since I was twelve, my mom
was standing out front, tending to the garden. She opened the
van's door and helped me to my feet. "*Mon dieu,*" she said, hand
over mouth, when she got a good look at me. "Why didn't you tell
me it was this bad?"

"It's a new 'heroin-chic' look I'm trying," I replied. My mom,
whose deranged sense of humor I could usually count on, did not
laugh.

"You haven't seen the worst of it," my dad said. "Sus, show her
your mouth."

I pulled down my bottom lip, wincing as I exposed three new
sores, milky full moons, round and swollen, that had cropped up
during the flight. My parents exchanged a look I couldn't deci-
pher.

Shuffling into the house, I went straight up the front stairs and
into my bedroom, my shoulders sagging with relief as I inhaled
the familiar scent of dusty books and spied the yellowing poster
of the legendary Tunisian singer Ali Riahi tacked to the wall. I
sprawled onto the bed, a heavy sleep pinning me to the mattress.
Hours passed and I woke up to the sound of the Swiss cowbell
that my mother rang to call everyone down for dinner—a nod to
her roots, and a source of profound irritation to my brother and
me. I stoppered my ears, trying to fall back asleep. When I didn't
answer, my dad appeared, knocking at my door.

"*Labess?*" he asked, Tunisian slang for What's going on?

"Not hungry," I groaned, pulling the pillow over my head.

"It's been months since we've seen you. At least come sit with us for a bit."

"I'm too tired," I said.

"You've been sleeping for hours. You need to make more of an effort. You'll feel better once you're up. Come on, let's eat and go for a walk around the block."

"Hédi. *Please.*"

I lay motionless for a while after my father gave up and left, a mixture of guilt and doubt preventing me from falling back asleep. I knew something was wrong, but there were still moments when I wondered if I was making it all up—if my symptoms were real or only in my head. Maybe I did just need to make more of an effort.

I got out of bed and made my way to the landing at the top of the staircase. The steps seemed to go on forever as I slogged down, my limbs heavy containers filled with cement. When I reached the bottom, I was so depleted I sank to the oak floor and tried to regain my strength. I could hear the sound of my parents' voices in the kitchen. I cocked an ear, the old childhood instinct to eavesdrop too tempting to resist.

"I let her buy a return ticket to Paris for two weeks from now, but I doubt she'll be well enough to go," my mom said. "Not anytime soon."

"What do you think of when you hear the symptoms: mouth sores, weight loss, frequent infections, and low blood counts?" asked my dad.

My mom was silent.

"HIV," he said, sounding like he had given this some thought. "I know the test results came back negative, but I read online that it can take several months for the virus to show up. Did you see how much she and her friends were drinking at graduation? And that was in front of us. Who knows what she's been up to when we're not there. She could be sleeping around or using drugs, for all we know."

My face was on fire. A bolt of adrenaline shot to my chest, and I ran up the stairs, pulse racing, trembling hands slamming my bedroom door shut. I was furious at my father for speculating about the state of my health and my character behind my back. I felt a deep shame, too. He wasn't entirely mistaken; my life away from home had involved some of the things he feared. But what rattled me most was that my father, who always fronted as tough, sounded scared for me. It was becoming harder to believe the line I'd been fed since I was a kid: *Everything is going to be all right.*

6

BIFURCATION

A WEEK HAD passed since my return home. I remember only dimly how I spent the time. I went to a flurry of doctors' appointments, I slept a lot, and I skyped with Will. I reluctantly dragged myself out for walks around the block with my parents. But what I remember most is the anxious hush that had fallen over the household; the worry that filled the air; the mounting fear and frustration I felt as I waited for clarity.

Today was Easter, but I ruined it, I wrote in my journal. *Anne spent 6 hours preparing an incredible meal for dad and me. Not only did I eat nothing, but all I could do was stare glumly at the two of them. On Wednesday I am scheduled to have a bone marrow biopsy and I am dreading it.*

"Precautionary" was the word the doctor used when he suggested the biopsy. It was a torturous, humiliating procedure that entailed lying facedown on an examining room table with my jeans around my ankles. The doctor cleaned my lower back with Betadine as he explained that the pelvic bone, rich in marrow, was the preferred location for the biopsy. He injected lidocaine into my lower back, plunging the needle deeper and deeper until it struck bone. Although the surface layers of my skin were numb, it would still hurt, the doctor warned. I gritted my teeth as he slid a thin syringe into the bone and aspirated the marrow cells with quick nauseating sucks. Next came a much bigger needle—ten inches of gleaming stainless steel—with a plastic handle at the top that he would use to drill deeper into the marrow. My bones were young and strong, the doctor said, as he put one shoe up on the exam table, grunting as he bore down into my pelvic bone. As he clipped off a small, solid chunk of marrow, I bit the inside of my cheek, tasting blood. Once the procedure was over, I sat there dazed with a big bandage covering the biopsy site, my back throbbing. The doctor reassured me that he didn't expect to find anything abnormal, but given my worsening condition, he wanted to take every precaution.

A week later, on May 3, 2011, we received a message on the answering machine. The preliminary results of the biopsy were in, and the doctor wanted us to come in as soon as possible. By the time my parents and I arrived at the clinic, the staff and the other patients had gone home for the day. It was after hours and the lights in the office had been dimmed, casting shadows across the stacks of magazines and pea-green walls. The doctor came out to meet us in the waiting room and sat down. He didn't mince words. "The biopsy confirmed what I suspected but hoped wouldn't be the case. You have something called acute myeloid leukemia." He enunciated the diagnosis slowly, like a foreign-language instructor teaching us a new vocabulary word.

I didn't know what it meant, but I could tell it wasn't good. I averted my eyes from my parents' devastated faces. Frozen in my chair, I repeated the diagnosis over and over in my head. *Loo-kee-*

mee-ah. Loo-kee-mee-ah. Loo-kee-mee-ah. It sounded like an exotic flower, beautiful and poisonous.

"It's an aggressive form of cancer that attacks the blood and bone marrow," the doctor said, his shoulders drooping a little beneath his lab coat. "We'll need to act fast."

How do you react to a cancer diagnosis at age twenty-two?

Do you break down in sobs?

Do you faint, or scream?

In that moment, a feeling flooded through my body, unexpected and perverse: relief. After the bewildering months of misdiagnosis, I finally had an explanation for my itch, for my mouth sores, for my unraveling. I wasn't a hypochondriac, after all, making up symptoms. My fatigue was not evidence of partying too hard or an inability to cut it in the real world, but something concrete, something utterable that I could wrap my tongue around.

Everything the doctor said after—that the situation was grave and that I would need to begin treatment right away—faded into a distant hum. Instead, it felt as if he were standing over me with a scalpel, cleaving my life by diagnosis, bifurcating my psyche into separate selves: half of me dancing with a mariachi singer after tequila shots at Don Juan, a bar in Paris, making my friends whistle and cheer; half of me crying every night in a sterile hospital room after the visitors had gone home.

The diagnosis had formed an irreparable fracture: my life before, and after.

7

FALLOUT

A FAMILY OF public criers we are not. When we got home that
night, my mom retreated to her studio and closed the door; I
locked myself in my bedroom, curled into a fetal ball, and pulled
the covers over my head; my dad went for a long walk in the woods
near our house, returning several hours later with bloodshot eyes.
My brother, Adam, a junior in college, was studying abroad in
Argentina, and my parents and I decided to spare him the news of
my diagnosis until we knew more about what my treatment would
entail. As for my friends, they had no idea that I'd been unwell, or
that I was back in the United States; they were still posting on my
Facebook wall asking if they could visit me in Paris.

Lying on my bed, I felt an impulse to share my terrible news.
If I said it out loud, I thought it might begin to feel real. I picked
up the phone and rang Jake, one of my closest college friends. I
wanted practice before I tried to find the right words for Will, and
I trusted that Jake would understand—but to this day, I've never
heard anyone get off the phone so fast. He apologized, telling me

he wished he could talk longer but he had plans. He promised to call back later that night. He didn't. I wouldn't hear from him for many weeks. It was my first indication that cancer is uncomfortable for the people around you, and that when people don't know what to say, they often say nothing at all.

Before I lost what was left of my courage, I dialed Will. We were still in the early stages of our relationship. What did I expect? That he would drop everything and move again—that he would come here, to Saratoga, and live with me and my parents, whom he'd never even met? As the phone rang, I steeled myself with deep, gulping breaths. "The biopsy results came back. I have something called acute myeloid leukemia," I told him, my voice hoarse. "I have no idea what's going to happen. I know you didn't sign up for this."

I went on to explain what little I knew about my diagnosis and that I wouldn't be returning to Paris anytime soon. Home, for the foreseeable future, would be my childhood bedroom until I entered the hospital to begin chemotherapy. A second passed, maybe two, but the silence seemed like an eternity. I heard footsteps and the sound of a cupboard banging shut. It was morning in Paris, and I pictured him pacing around our apartment, with bed head and a cup of coffee in his hand. "I'm catching the first flight to New York," he said. "I'm on my way to the airport right now." It was only then that I began to cry.

Cancer is great gossip. Within twenty-four hours, word of my diagnosis swept through our small town like a fire through sagebrush. The light on the answering machine at my parents' house was blinking red: at full capacity. A message from a neighbor asking if the news was true and if so, how they could help. Another, from a childhood friend whom I hadn't seen in more than a decade, offering to visit. A colleague of my father's telling us that she would drop off a pot of chili for dinner. And confirmation from a man my family would come to call "the Cancer Guru" about an appointment that we had forgotten all about.

We had scheduled the appointment a few days before my diagnosis, because an acquaintance of my mother's from yoga said he was good at cracking medical mysteries. "Maybe he can offer some supplements to help you feel a little better," my mother said. It sounded reasonable. When my brother and I were growing up, she had taught us that fast food, soda, and sugary cereal were poison. The health food store, the acupuncturist, the Chinese herbalist, and the homeopath were always our first stops—a regular doctor's office was a last resort. As a kid, I had found my mother's obsession with health embarrassing. (On Halloween, she was the lady on the block who handed out unshelled peanuts, apples, and number two pencils instead of candy.) But over the years, I absorbed her commitment to alternative medicine and all things organic, and ultimately I came to see value in it.

A few hours later, I sat in the passenger's seat as my mother drove, watching the landmarks of my childhood blur past—the main drag of downtown Saratoga where I'd busked for crumpled dollar bills as a teenager, the used bookstore where I'd had my first kiss, the elementary school where I'd arrived as a kindergartner who didn't speak a word of English. We drove on, down two-lane country roads, until we arrived, forty-five minutes later, at a small, wooded trailer park on the outskirts of a town I had never heard of before. We pulled up to a double-wide, the grass littered with lawn ornaments, got out of the car, and knocked on the door.

A man with yellowish hair and a ponderous gut that draped over his blue jeans answered. My mother immediately shared with him the news of my diagnosis. Before I could take off my jacket, he clamped a meaty hand around my arm and leaned in, close enough that I could feel his dank breath on my cheek. "Before we begin, I want to make one thing very clear," he said, peering deep into my pupils. "You *will* die if you go forward with any traditional chemotherapy treatments."

The Cancer Guru explained that he would use a muscle-testing technique to get a clearer picture of what was going on. It entailed putting drops of various flower extracts onto my tongue and then assessing my body's strength in response. For the next hour, I stood like a scarecrow in the living room of the trailer, exchanging bewildered looks with my mother, as the Cancer Guru pushed down on my outstretched arms, fiddled with hundreds of little glass vials, and scribbled notes onto a piece of paper.

"You can sit now," he said finally. Exhausted, I sank into the couch next to my mother, both of us eager for the appointment to be over. But the Cancer Guru was just warming up. "I have good news and I have bad news," he told my mother. "The bad news is that your daughter does in fact have leukemia." He said it solemnly, as though there had been some doubt on the subject before. "The good news is that I can cure her."

The Cancer Guru then began to preach, stomping his feet and waving his hands for emphasis, like some coke-addled televangelist. Over the next hour and a half, he bombarded us with tale after tale of cancer patients who had ignored his advice and gone to the hospital for their treatments. "They never left!" he shouted in a thunderous voice. "They died agonizing, chemotherapy-induced deaths! Do you want that to happen to you? Do you?"

I wish I could say that my mother and I cut off the Cancer Guru—that we told him just where to put those glass vials of flower extract. But being afraid for your life can scramble the senses, can turn your tongue to chalk. As the Cancer Guru continued to hurl his theories at us, my mother and I shrank into the stained paisley pillows of the couch. It was only when he ushered us into the tiny kitchen at the front of the trailer and attempted to draw my blood with unwashed hands that my mother dropped her fist on the table, and said, in a trembling voice, "I think it's time for us to go." We put on our coats and left, but only after he pressured us into buying two hundred dollars' worth of vitamin supplements and several gallons of aloe vera juice on our way out.

On the drive home, my mom and I sat in stunned silence. "I can't believe I put you through that," she said. "I feel like the worst mother in the world. I'm so sorry, so, so sorry—"

Later I would come to see this incident—and so many others along the surreal journey of contending with cancer—as darkly comic. But in the moment, I was weighted heavily with a sense of responsibility. It had only been forty-eight hours, but already my diagnosis had overturned our lives, yanking us all through a trapdoor into this strange, confusing land.

So before my mother could finish, I cut in. "It's my fault. I'm the one who got us into this whole mess in the first place."

Back home, in the safety of my bedroom, I turned full investigative reporter. After twenty minutes of Internet sleuthing, I discovered that the Cancer Guru was not in fact a trained kinesiologist, as he had claimed, but a veterinarian. A decade earlier, he had been arraigned on a seventy-one-count indictment for unlicensed practice of medicine and dentistry on the wrong species: humans. One of the charges detailed how he had used dirty needles to inject patients with urine. These allegations followed an earlier investigation in 1995 that found him guilty of unauthorized medical practice after he advised a patient to drink three gallons of water and consume a hundred supplements a day, resulting in the woman being hospitalized.

Going forward, I vowed to learn everything I could about my diagnosis: burying my head in research journals, making a list of experts to interview, scouring every corner of the Internet for information. I needed to find a way to take control of what was happening to me, and I decided that the more I could glean about my disease, the greater my chances of survival. *Knowledge is power,* right? But as I dug into my new disease over the next few hours, I didn't feel empowered. The statistics I stumbled across turned my blood to ice. The chill deepened as I learned that only one in four patients with my type of leukemia survived five years past diagnosis. I wondered if my parents knew this. I prayed they didn't.

Forty-eight hours after my diagnosis, I watched from behind the curtains of my bedroom window as a car pulled up, tires crunching on the gravel driveway. Will was here, fresh off the plane from Paris. He paused on the sidewalk to take in the leafy, tree-lined block and the white Victorian with green shutters, flanked by the lilac bushes, daffodils, and bleeding hearts my mother tended to each afternoon. For a moment, I wasn't sure what made me more nervous: Will meeting my parents for the first time or the chemo I was scheduled to begin in a few days. In the past, my father had always been unsparingly tough on my boyfriends—though it might be more accurate to say that he barely acknowledged their existence. But this time, it was different. When he met Will, he shook his hand and kept thanking him for coming. "I'm so glad you're here," my father said.

For the first time, my parents did not make up the futon in the study when a boy came over to stay. I suppose we all had bigger problems to worry about now than keeping up appearances. It was humid and hot when Will and I went to bed that night, the air pushing down on us like a wet, wool blanket. We undressed and had sex in my childhood bedroom with its pink walls and posters, careful not to wake up my parents in the room next door. Afterward, Will began to weep. "A lot of bad things are about to happen," he said. "We need to put our relationship into a box and to protect it with everything we have."

8

DAMAGED GOODS

MY MOTHER, A talented classical pianist, taught me my first scales and started me on lessons in kindergarten, but it wasn't until the fourth grade that I chose music for myself. Miss McNamara, the music teacher at Lake Avenue Elementary School, stood in front of the class with a dozen stringed instruments lined up at the front of the room. "Come up and pick your instrument," she invited us.

The thought that I could choose my instrument was a revelation. The violins and cellos were the hottest items, but I was curious about the big wooden object at the end of the row, leaning up against the chalkboard. The double bass. It was taller than I was—taller than Richard Saxton, the tallest boy in my class—and what's more, my teacher told me I was one of the only girls in her memory who'd expressed interest in playing it. I felt strangely drawn to the instrument's bulk, its shapely wooden torso and long neck that curved heavenward into a scroll. I plucked at its strings, thick as worms, a low, pleasant grumble of notes emanating from the *f*-shaped holes. With my unpronounceable name and immigrant parents I'd always felt like a misfit at school, and the bass struck me as its own kind of outlier in the orchestra. That afternoon I took the instrument home and gave it a name: Charlie Brown. I was going to be a double bassist. "Okay fine," my mom said, "as long as you promise to keep up with your piano lessons."

At age sixteen, I was offered a scholarship to attend the precollege program at the Juilliard School in New York City. Every Saturday for the next two years, I rose at four in the morning, and my dad drove me the forty-five minutes to Albany so that I could catch the train to the city—a three-hour ride on Amtrak—often barely making it on time to my nine o'clock music theory class. After a long day of orchestra rehearsals, master classes, and auditions, I hauled my bass onto the M66 bus and rode across town to the Upper East Side, where I stayed the night with my friend Caroline and her family, then took the train back home the next morning. Everywhere I went, my bass came with me. It attracted stares— and sometimes unwanted offers of help from strange men. Lugging it around the subways and buses and sidewalks of Manhattan was a chore—especially for a teenage girl who insisted on wearing impractical shoes—but it was worth it. When I showed up somewhere to play, I felt like I had already warmed up.

Six years later, in the days after my diagnosis, I found myself making the same four-hour commute to the city and crashing at the same friend's house that I had as a teenager. But now I was on my way to meet with my new medical team. The doctor in Saratoga had said my leukemia was too advanced to be treated locally and that I would need to transfer my care to one of the cancer centers in Manhattan.

Caroline's father was a two-time cancer survivor and, upon hearing the news of my illness, had immediately called my parents to offer his support. He referred us to one of the city's most renowned oncologists and generously insisted that we stay at their apartment for as long as needed. This was all an extraordinary privilege, I would soon realize. Without the health insurance I received through my father's employer, the disability payments from my paralegal job that helped foot the already mounting medical bills, and the friends who offered us their home and their connections, my family would have faced financial ruin, and I, certain death.

Everything in Mount Sinai's cancer wing was baby-food beige: beige carpets, beige walls, beige vinyl chairs. The waiting room was crowded with patients, many of whom were bald, some in wheelchairs, others shuffling around with walkers. My parents and Will had come with me to this first appointment, and as we took a seat, I couldn't help but notice that I was the youngest patient by several decades in the room. There was a freezer by the reception desk with free ice cream, a thoughtful touch, and I helped myself to a strawberry popsicle. The ice numbed the half dozen sores that scourged the inside of my mouth. A television flickered from the corner of the waiting room, the sound on mute. On the screen I noticed a familiar face, a voluptuous blonde who was demonstrating how to make a watermelon and feta salad, adorned with sprigs of mint. I recognized her. She had been a year ahead of me at college and was now, apparently, hosting a cooking show on daytime television. Oh, and she also appeared to be pregnant—a round baby bump protruded beneath her apron. How strange to be here, in this depressing room, I thought with incredulity, while my peers were out there, starting careers, having babies, traveling the world, and hitting all the other milestones of young adulthood.

After almost two hours of waiting, we were escorted to a sterile room, where we were greeted by an older man wearing a white lab coat and a blue silk cravat. "I'm Dr. Holland," the man said, with a broad, warm smile. He had neatly combed white hair, bushy eyebrows, and a prominent nose. Although his back was stooped with age, he possessed a magisterial presence. "Rule number one: no hand shaking, with anyone," he instructed sternly, leaving my outstretched arm hanging. "Your low blood counts make you extremely vulnerable to germs, and you need to be very careful from now on."

Dr. Holland was the chief oncology officer of Mount Sinai Hospital. He was considered a founding father of chemotherapy and had helped pioneer lifesaving treatments for countless cancer patients. In the 1950s, when he finished medical school, leukemia was still considered a death sentence. He and his collaborators had been called "research cowboys" by their colleagues for attempting to treat the incurable disease with several chemotherapy drugs simultaneously instead of sequentially. The clinical trial to contain leukemia that Dr. Holland directed had proved successful, and had since become the standard treatment for patients like me. Now, despite being in his late eighties, he still worked five days a week, both seeing patients and conducting research. His eyes, magnified by enormous wire-rimmed glasses, missed nothing, as he studied me and my entourage. "You must be the mother and father," he said, nodding at my parents. "And you are?" he asked, turning to Will.

"The boyfriend," Will replied.

"Very good. I'm glad to see you all here," Dr. Holland said. "Suleika is going to need your support, a lot of it. And you are going to need to take good care of yourselves so that you can be strong for her."

Over the next half hour, Dr. Holland prepared us for what was to come as my mother dutifully took notes. I would be admitted to the hospital tomorrow or the day after, and I would stay for roughly three weeks, as I underwent an aggressive course of chemotherapy. The goal was to get rid of as many of the leukemia cells—or "blast cells," in medical jargon—as possible. These large, immature, rapidly multiplying monsters signified the presence of cancer in my bone marrow. The chemo regimen, referred to as "seven plus three," consisted of two highly potent intravenous drugs, cytarabine and daunorubicin, which I would receive for seven days. All these new terms were overwhelming, and I found myself wishing I'd paid better attention in my high school science classes. "If all goes well, you'll be home recuperating before you know it and you can enjoy the rest of summer," he said optimistically, while being careful not to make any promises.

Dr. Holland asked me to hop up on the exam table. He looked in my mouth, clucking his tongue at the sores, and made a note to prescribe something stronger for my pain. He listened to my heart and lungs and palpated my hollowed abdomen. Midway through the exam, we were interrupted by two doctors, a middle-aged man with a gray mustache and a young woman with long, dangly emerald earrings. "Sorry to interrupt," one of them said. "The rest of her biopsy results just came in, and we need you to take a look right away." All three doctors scurried out of the room, leaving us alone. Will, my parents, and I sat wordlessly, exchanging worried glances.

When they returned a few minutes later, Dr. Holland's mouth was drawn into a flat, grim hyphen. He explained that further test results had revealed that my leukemia was far more complicated than anyone could have predicted. I had a rare bone marrow disorder called myelodysplastic syndrome, known as pre-leukemia, that had gone undiagnosed. I'd likely had it for a long time, which explained the slow onslaught of symptoms I'd experienced over the last year—the itch, the exhaustion, the anemia, the shortness of breath, and the frequent colds—before my condition had grown more acute and turned into full-fledged leukemia. Myelodysplastic syndrome typically affected patients older than sixty, Dr. Holland explained. It had no known cause, although it was linked to exposure to toxic chemicals like benzene, pesticides, and heavy metals like lead.

"When you were a baby, I used to take you to my studio and I painted with you strapped to my chest in a sling," my mother said, her face stiff with guilt. "Is it possible that exposure to the paint fumes caused this?"

"This is no one's fault," Dr. Holland said gently. "Sometimes these things just happen, and we don't know why. You mustn't blame yourself."

Up until this point, the extent of my knowledge about bone marrow came from French cuisine—*boeuf à la moelle*, the fancy dish occasionally served with a side of toasted baguette. Dr. Holland explained that the marrow, an organ at the very core of the body, was a living, sponge-like tissue that filled almost every bone. In a healthy person, the marrow was responsible for producing all of the body's blood cells: white cells that fight off infection, red cells that provide oxygen, and platelets that stanch bleeding. In a person with myelodysplastic syndrome, the process was disrupted; instead of developing normally, the blood cells died in the bone marrow or just after entering the bloodstream. Even with extensive chemotherapy, I would eventually go into something called "bone marrow failure." Other ominous terms I didn't understand yet like "multiple chromosomal abnormalities," "monosomy seven," and "poor prognosis" were also mentioned.

All this meant that, in addition to chemo, I would eventually need a bone marrow transplant. It was a dangerous, complicated procedure with a high mortality rate, but it was my only shot at a cure, Dr. Holland explained. I would be eligible for transplant only if the chemo managed to reduce the percentage of leukemic blasts in my marrow to under 5 percent—and, of course, if I was able to find a suitable donor. Without a donor, the path to a cure became much less certain, or even impossible. Finding a match was especially challenging for minorities who were underrepresented in bone marrow registries. As a first-generation American from a mixed ethnic background, I found myself in a scary place.

A harried, global search for a Swiss-Tunisian bone marrow match would delay the process. My brother, who was still studying abroad in Argentina, was my best hope. He would need to leave school and fly back to New York right away to be tested. But Dr. Holland was careful to temper hope with reality. Siblings were the best chance for a match, but a match only happened about 25 percent of the time. I had thought that receiving a diagnosis meant an end to the months of uncertainty. I was wrong. Medicine, I was learning, was more of an art than a science in cases like mine.

Dr. Holland sighed, looking very tired all of a sudden. "We have a long, difficult road ahead. Leukemia is a young doctor's disease and I won't be able to handle your case alone. I'm assigning Dr. Navada and Dr. Silverman to help with your care," he said, gesturing to his colleagues. "Together, we'll work as a team to make sure you receive the very best treatment. We promise to do everything we can to help you make it to the other side."

Later that night, I lay in the dark, not sleeping. It was three in the morning and Will was snoring lightly beside me. I opened my laptop and began to read up on the bone marrow transplant process, as well as the chemo regimen I was slated to start in a few days. There, on the list of side effects, sandwiched between vomiting, hair loss, heart damage, and organ failure, I saw something that upset me more than any of the bad news I'd received so far: The cancer treatment that could save my life would also most likely leave me infertile. Since my diagnosis, I had felt relief, followed by shock, confusion, and horror. And now, something else: a wrenching sense of foreclosing.

Cancer is an emergency, and oncologists are the first responders: They are trained to beat it, and everything else must take a backseat. But no one on my medical team, as the treatment plan was drawn up, had mentioned infertility as a potential side effect. It was only after I asked about infertility at our appointment the next day that my oncologists told me about the available options: I could undergo fertility preservation treatments, freezing either my eggs or embryos. Depending on where I was in my menstrual cycle, this could take several weeks, and I would have to delay chemo, which they strongly advised against. But ultimately the choice was mine.

As much as I appreciated their support, the absence of communication on something so important felt like a breach of trust early on in our patient-doctor relationship. Most patients afflicted with my type of leukemia were long past their childbearing years. While my medical team was intent on saving my life, preserving my chance to be a mother someday hadn't seemed to be on their radar. It was my first indication that, no matter how brilliant and compassionate my doctors might be, I would have to be proactive and learn to advocate for myself.

At twenty-two years old, the most thought I'd ever given to motherhood was how not to become a mother before I was ready. The few times I'd had reason to buy a pregnancy test in college, I remembered the rush of relief I'd felt, sitting in my dorm room, as only one line, not two, appeared on the stick. But now, as I considered the possibility of never being able to have my own children, my throat tightened with grief. I had always secretly thought that if I did get pregnant when I was older it would happen the way it had for my mother: organically and unplanned, but a welcome surprise. No longer.

After the appointment with my oncologists, I walked with my family and Will to a nearby restaurant for lunch. Everywhere I looked, the sidewalks seemed to be teeming with pregnant women, young mothers wheeling around newborns in prams and children in school uniforms skipping and singing as they walked home. Watching them, I felt a wave of yearning, some primordial part of me rising up. While I still wasn't sure if I wanted kids, I knew in this moment that I wanted to do everything in my power to keep this option open for my future self.

The family minivan idled at the intersection of Fifty-ninth and York. Will swabbed my midriff with alcohol as he steadied the needle. My parents looked on from the front seat, quietly studying the young man they had known for a little over two weeks. The needle was filled with gonadotropin, a hormone that stimulates the ovaries to produce eggs. A nurse at the fertility clinic had taught us how to administer the injections on a flesh-colored cushion. Because I was terrified of needles, either Will or my mother had helped administer the shots each morning and night for the past ten days, pinching the skin on my abdomen, injecting it with the vials of medication. Here at the end of our drive from Saratoga to Manhattan, Will was taking his turn.

Traffic was at a standstill, and we were late for my last appointment at the fertility clinic. The atmosphere was tense. As soon as the fertility treatments were done, I would have to enter the hospital and begin chemo, and I wouldn't be able to return home for several weeks. The evening before, I sat at the table in my parents' backyard as my dad cooked calamari on the grill with a spicy, harissa-infused sauce, his childhood favorite. My mom lit candles and Will helped set the table. I should have been savoring my last days of freedom, but I was agitated from the fertility drugs. They made me moody and bloated, the waistband of my jeans straining against my bruised stomach. I looked across the table at Will. We had only been together for six months, but there we were with my parents, discussing the pros and cons of freezing embryos versus freezing only my eggs. By every objective measure, it was awkward territory.

"I'm putting my life at risk by delaying the chemo," I said. "I've committed to doing this fertility thing, so I think I should go the embryo route since it's got a greater chance of success."

"But to make embryos, you need . . . *sperm,*" my mother said, her Swiss accent wrapping strangely around the word.

"I was thinking I could get a donor, like, from a sperm bank."

"Really?" she asked. "You wouldn't necessarily know who the donor is, what he's like, where he's from, what his family medical history might—"

"I'm the one who's damaged goods here," I snapped. This came out harsher than I meant it, and my mother looked as if she might cry. My father's eyes stayed focused on the squid, the conversation having long departed his comfort zone.

Turning to me, Will said, "I could be your sperm donor. I know how much this means to you, but, of course, it's up to you."

In this moment, I loved him more deeply than I knew it possible to love anyone. I loved that he had shown up for me during the worst week of my life. I loved that he'd immediately gotten along with my parents and was always finding ways to make us all laugh, despite the awful circumstances in which we'd come together. And I loved that he was willing to delve into the difficult subjects—of eggs and sperm and embryos, of my future children, maybe even *our* future children, and how they could be brought into the world. I loved, too, that he was man enough to talk about all this in front of my father, rather than fleeing for the nearest exit.

Inside the fertility clinic, the walls were bare except for a sign that said: NO CHILDREN ALLOWED. Several women, some alone, others with partners, sat in plush chairs, waiting for the lady in the lab coat to call the next name. I guessed that most of the women were paying full price to be here. Fertility preservation treatments could cost upward of twenty-five thousand dollars and were often not covered by insurance. In my case, my medical team had helped me secure a grant through an organization called Fertile Hope to cover the bill.

In most doctors' offices, it is hard to know why the stranger next to you is there, but everyone was here for the same reason. The room was tense. No one was talking, but everybody seemed to be sizing one another up. Most of the women appeared to be in their mid-thirties, and a few might have been in their forties. Based on how they were dressed, I guessed they had jobs to return to after their appointments. As I sat there, with my parents and boyfriend, wearing my college hoodie emblazoned with CLASS OF 2010, I felt profoundly out of place.

A nurse called me into the exam room. She drew my blood to test my estrogen levels, then gave me a cup of apple juice to sip. Then I stripped off my clothes and dressed in a cotton gown. I lay on the table, the tissue paper crinkling beneath me as I nestled my feet into the metal stirrups. The fertility doctor, a man with dyed black hair, placed a large rubbery condom onto a transvaginal ultrasound wand. I cringed as I heard the squish of lube being squeezed onto the end of the knob and shut my eyes as it nosed its way in between my legs. The doctor switched on the monitor, searching my ovaries until my follicles, the fluid-filled sacs where the eggs mature, appeared, resembling a honeycomb. "Congratulations, it looks like you're ripe for harvesting," the doctor said, nodding at the screen. "Have you decided if you want to create embryos or to freeze only your eggs?"

"As of right now, I'm thinking embryos," I said. "My boyfriend, Will, has offered to be my sperm donor."

"I see," the doctor replied evenly. "In that case I think it would be a good idea for the two of you to meet with the social worker before you leave so that you can fill out the necessary paperwork."

My eggs, or "totsicles" as Will and I had started to refer to them, would be surgically removed the next day. I would undergo anesthesia, and the procedure, which the doctor assured me should be quick and mostly painless, would last no more than half an hour. The eggs would then be fertilized with sperm in a petri dish to form embryos and stored in a cryobank.

A few minutes later, the social worker summoned Will and me into her office. She cautioned us strongly against the embryos, citing the unforeseeable legal and emotional obstacles that could arise down the road: *How could we plan to have a child when we had only recently started dating? What if we broke up? And what would happen if I didn't survive—who would own the embryos then?* As I tried to formulate a counterargument, I came up empty. Will sat silently, his head bent low, staring at his shoes. I had put off the decision for as long as I could. Now the fertility doctor was back, waiting for my answer, but I was swarmed by questions of my own: *How could I possibly make such a choice in such a short amount of time? How could I choose between the hope I had for our future together and the undeniable fact that nothing was guaranteed? Between the headiness of new love and the chilly stringency of logic?* The seconds ticked by, and finally, I had to give an answer. With more than a little reluctance, I told the doctor to freeze only my eggs.

The timing of all this, like everything else in recent days, felt hopelessly out of sequence. But this was my new reality. As far as I knew, the women in the waiting room didn't have cancer, but I was linked to them. My breasts, like theirs, were tender and swollen from the hormone injections. Our bodies were sending us signals to get ready for pregnancy even though none of us could be certain it would happen. Although I wasn't planning for a baby anytime soon, preserving my ability to have one felt like my only lifeline to an uncertain future.

9

BUBBLE GIRL

IT WAS A perfect spring morning on the Upper East Side of Manhattan, the sky a crisp, vivid blue. We parked the minivan and walked the ten blocks to Mount Sinai Hospital, passing the parade of uniformed doormen along Fifth Avenue. I noticed the clouds floating flimsily overhead like tissue paper. I noticed Central Park, bursting with color, the luscious greens of young leaves sprouting from trees, the fuchsia spray of azalea bushes, the pale yellow tulips shooting up from the earth. I opened my eyes wider, trying to take it all in, to memorize the feel of the sun on my hair, the way the spring air breezed the nape of my neck.

When we reached the steps at the hospital's main entrance, my parents stopped to give me a silver necklace with a turquoise charm. "For each new milestone you reach in your treatment, I'll give you another charm," my mother said, her mouth smiling but her eyes frosting over with a sadness I hadn't seen before. Will, too, had a gift, and he handed me a purple Moleskine notebook. Inside, under "In case of loss please return to:" he had written my childhood nickname "Susu" and "$1,000,000 reward if returned to the owner." As we opened the glass doors and stepped inside, I took one last gulp of fresh air, bottling it in my lungs for as long as I could, knowing it would be a long time before I would be allowed outside again.

I was escorted upstairs to the oncology ward and put into a drab room with stark white walls and two hospital beds. Both were empty, so I chose the one closest to the window. I hung up my favorite summer dress in the closet like an athlete retiring a jersey and changed into a backless hospital gown. An electronic bracelet was strapped to my right wrist, a precaution against patients who, drugged to the gills on painkillers or lost in a fog of dementia, sometimes tried to wander out of the hospital. I signed so many forms I lost count, including one that designated my mother as my healthcare proxy. I also filled out an advance directive. Then, I was wheeled off to surgery, where they implanted a catheter in my chest, creating a central line through which chemo and intravenous fluids would be administered.

When I woke up in the surgical recovery room, I looked down at my bloodied chest. Protruding from a wound below my collarbone, I saw a plastic tube with three dangling lumens, like the tentacles of some abhorrent sea creature. The sight of my altered body shocked me. I leaned over the handrails of the gurney and vomited. Up until this moment, with the exception of the mouth sores, my illness had been largely invisible. On some level, I was starting to realize that the life I'd had before was shattered—the person I'd been, buried. I would never be the same. Even my name had been changed, if only inadvertently. As I was wheeled back to the oncology ward I noticed that the sign outside my hospital room read S. JAQUAD—with a *q* where the *o* should be. I was crossing over into a new land. And with every step I was feeling less like Suleika.

Two nurses entered my room carrying IV bags of antinausea medications and chemo that would drip through my veins for the next week. The younger nurse introduced herself as Younique. She looked to be about my age, and her hair, jet-black and hot-combed, was tied back into a serviceable knot. I eyed her with the skeptical air of someone who is about to allow herself to be poisoned by a perfect stranger. "Watch out for that little guy," Younique warned, pointing to the smaller of the two bags. It contained one of the chemo drugs and was the color of fruit punch. "Some call it the Red Devil because its side effects can be gnarly. Anything you need, just ring the call button."

Will and my parents sat on folding chairs, watching me until the sun went from hot white to a dusky orange outside the window. I filled the silences with dumb jokes and a steady stream of mindless chitchat. I'd brought my slippers and my favorite stuffed animal from home, as well as a stack of books that I intended to work my way through during my time in the hospital. "I feel like I just moved into a dorm room on the first day of college," I said enthusiastically, picking up Tolstoy's *War and Peace* and flipping the pages. "I'll be able to catch up on reading. Maybe I can even get some writing done while I'm here."

I meant what I said—I did want to charge forward, to try to accomplish something. I'd been operating on a bizarre high since my diagnosis, adrenaline and fear charging my body, a desperate optimism coursing through my arteries. The deadly disease tearing through my blood and marrow, the spartan sadness of this hospital room, the terrifying side effects of the chemo that lay ahead—I was certain none of it would break me. If anything, this experience would make me stronger. Who knew? I might even become one of those former cancer patients who go on to start a research foundation or to run ultramarathons. But mostly I wanted to ease the worry clouding my parents' and Will's faces—to convince them I was going to be okay. They smiled weakly at me, murmuring words of encouragement, as I blabbered on.

Eventually the sky darkened. "Go home and get some rest," I told my parents and Will, who were staying at our family friend's apartment a few blocks away. They looked exhausted but didn't budge. Only when I insisted did they stand up to leave. "Are you sure you'll be all right on your own?" my mom asked, lingering by the door. "I'm great," I said cheerfully, waving them off.

It was only after they left that the brave face I'd been wearing all day began to crumple and fold.

Oncology wards, more than maybe anywhere on earth, are music-less places. Instead of flowing melody, there's incessant beeping. During the day, the halls clamor with a constant medical call-and-response loop: nurses hollering to one another; patients calling, sometimes screaming, for morphine; nurses scrambling to find doctors; visitors searching frantically for nurses. But in some ways, those noises—however annoying—are a welcome distraction, a reminder that the hospital "machine" is in healthy operation. It is the quiet hours after dark, the hollow sounds of silent suffering, that are most frightening.

Younique had given me an Ambien before bed. Within minutes I fell into a heavy slumber, dragged into a hole darker than night as I dreamed of all the patients before me who had shared my same hospital pillow, their gaunt faces flashing through my sleep. Groggy and disoriented, I woke up around 2:00 A.M., the sound of whimpering rousing me from my nightmares. At first, I thought I might be hallucinating, but when I turned on the light, I discovered I had a roommate, a woman in her seventies who had arrived in the night. Her eyes were squeezed shut, mouth twisted in agony, as she panted short and fast through cracked lips. She moaned, tossing and turning in a drugged stupor. The presence of this stranger, submerged in her pain, gave me a glimpse of what lay ahead. I clicked off the light and pulled the gauzy green curtain between our beds shut, not wanting to see any more. I closed my eyes, trying to summon the strength and optimism I'd felt earlier in the day. Instead I found only terror.

As quietly as I could, I picked up the phone and dialed Will's number. "What's wrong?" he asked, his voice felted with sleep. I tried to speak but no sound emerged from my throat. "I'm hopping into a cab, I'll be right there," he said.

Half an hour later, his lanky silhouette filled the doorway. He tiptoed past my new roommate to my side of the room and wriggled in beside me, his long legs extending over the edge of my hospital bed. "What happens when NBA players get cancer? Do they have to order custom-made, extra-long hospital beds?" I whispered. "Good question," Will replied. "Let's just be glad you're the patient." I scooted up to the top of the mattress so that we lay forehead to forehead. I relaxed into Will, going slack in his arms, breathing in his warm, soapy scent, like a bundle of clothes fresh out of the dryer.

When I woke up the next morning, my roommate was in much better spirits. "Yo, Park Avenue!" she called out as I walked to the joint bathroom that was located on her side of the room. It was my fifth trip that morning—the egg retrieval surgery had left me with a painful urinary tract infection.

"Hi," I said, leaning against my IV pole. "I'm Suleika; it's really nice to meet you."

"Estelle," she replied, waving from her bed. "Pleasure."

"Why'd you call me Park Avenue?"

"Because you've got that fancy hairdo."

My hand traveled self-consciously to the freshly cut, chin-length bob framing my jaw. A few days before entering the hospital I'd asked a hairdresser to shear off my waist-length mane. A preemptive strike against the chemo that would soon claim all of my hair as its prize.

"I used to have it long," I explained to Estelle. "Thought I'd shave my head before coming here, but my mom said she wasn't ready to see me like that. So, I compromised." The hairdresser had given me my shorn hair to take home, a long auburn braid, which I'd asked my mother to donate to Locks of Love. Months later I'd find it in a small wooden jewelry box, tucked away in her studio.

"Well, I think you look real nice, but I'm going to keep calling you Park Avenue if that's all right," Estelle said. "I've got a bad case of chemo brain, and I know I won't be able to remember that other name of yours."

I laughed, nodding. "What brings you here?" I wanted to ask her what type of cancer she had, but I wasn't yet sure what the etiquette was between patients.

"Liver cancer, stage four. What about you? A young lady like yourself shouldn't be here. You should be out and about with your man. That's right, don't think I didn't hear you two last night!"

I blushed. "Leukemia, stage . . . I don't know. I haven't asked the doctors yet."

"Surgery? Radiation? Chemo?" Estelle asked, as though we were discussing Italian soda flavors.

"Chemo, my first round. They say I'll be here for three weeks or so."

"Ooph, that's a long one. Better go walk around the unit and get some exercise while you still can."

Per Estelle's advice, I got in the habit of seizing the moments when I had enough energy to explore. Using my IV pole as a makeshift skateboard, I zipped around the cancer ward, chatting up the nurses and the other patients; within a few days, I'd made a handful of friends. "Oncology's tween queen," Will crowned me in jest. A year too old for pediatrics but decades younger than most of the other patients in adult oncology, I felt out of place, but I was trying to make the best of the circumstances.

It was during one of my skateboarding sessions that I met Dennis, who was in his early forties and never seemed to have any visitors. When our meal trays kept arriving with the food still frozen—some genius forgetting to nuke them in the microwave—Dennis declared a hunger strike, going door to door to rally the other patients. I was all for hospital activism, but I was also concerned for his health. After a day or two, I asked Will to go find him the frothiest chocolate milkshake the Upper East Side had to offer, promptly bringing the hunger strike to an end.

In the room next to mine was a woman who was always asleep. I caught glimpses of her curled in bed whenever I walked by. She was so skeletal she looked almost cadaverous, her skin a waxy, jaundiced hue. On most days, her teenage daughter came to visit. Then, one afternoon, I heard a low, strangled cry, an animal bellow of grief that pierced the wall between our rooms. I got out of bed and watched from my door as the nurses escorted the daughter down the hall, consoling her as she sobbed. Soon after, the mother's lifeless corpse was wheeled away and a custodian arrived to clean the room. By noon the next day, another patient had taken her place.

My new neighbor was from Algeria. His name was Yehya, and he was undergoing treatment for lymphoma. He had a distended belly, lymph nodes like overripe plums bulging from his neck, and the skinniest legs I'd ever seen. We quickly became pals, chatting away in a patois of French and Arabic about our fatherlands and faith and how lucky we were to have gotten sick in America, where we had access to this kind of medical care. It was Ramadan and his wife came to the hospital each night, carrying a giant Tupperware filled with *iftar*—the meal Muslims eat at sundown to break fast—but he rarely took more than a bite.

One day, the doctors moved Yehya to a private room, a few doors down, with a window overlooking Central Park. He wept with gratitude and dropped to his knees to pray, but accidentally fell and hit his head on the linoleum floor. "What happened?" the nurses shouted when they heard the crash, rushing in and ordering a CT scan of his brain. Later, Yehya confessed to me that he had lied to the nurses and told them he tripped. "I didn't want to seem like some kind of Muslim nut," he told me. Illness complicated everything, even—maybe, especially—prayer.

It had been roughly a week since I'd entered the hospital and started chemotherapy. I was feeling relatively fine, even spritely in comparison with the other patients on my floor, many of whom were bedridden or needed wheelchairs to get around. While it would be a stretch to say I was *enjoying* my hospital stay, I wasn't miserable, either. When I wasn't hanging out with the other inhabitants of the ward, Will and I played countless games of Scrabble. My parents visited me every day, spoiling me with little gifts and home-cooked dishes. And as word of my diagnosis got out, friends trickled in as well, bearing bouquets of flowers. I felt suspended— for the first time in my life, no one expected anything of me. I had the liberty to pass the time as I wanted. I wrote in my journal and signed up for an arts and crafts class. A hospital volunteer was teaching me how to knit and I was making a scarf that I planned to give to Will.

Naïvely, maybe even a little arrogantly, I began to think I'd been spared the more treacherous side effects of the chemo. Other than the usual fatigue and the mouth sores, I felt no different. Each morning, I examined my scalp in the mirror for signs that my hair was beginning to fall out, but it was thick and shiny, firmly rooted in its follicles. I thought I might be among the tiny percentage of patients who don't lose their hair during chemo and I regretted what now seemed like a hasty decision to chop it short. I even began to entertain the fantasy of moving into an apartment with Will once I was discharged. Maybe, come end of summer, I might be well enough to start working again.

Naïveté has a shelf life, however, and mine didn't last long.

About ten days in, I was moved into a private room—"isolation" the doctors called it—and forbidden from stepping outside under any circumstances. I hadn't known this was coming. I was shocked and a little pissed at the strict rules that accompanied my new digs but also relieved not to have a roommate. Anyone who entered my room, which I dubbed "the Bubble," had to wear the mandatory protective armor—face mask, gloves, surgical gown. My blood counts were being decimated by the chemo, my hemoglobin and platelets plummeting to dangerously low levels. Test results showed that I possessed nearly no white blood cells—*zero* the doctor on call said, cupping his hands into an O for emphasis. Soon I would be done with the chemo infusions, and over the next week, my marrow, hopefully now rid of leukemia, would start to recover and my blood cells would slowly build back up. Once I no longer needed transfusions to maintain my red blood cell and platelet counts, I would be discharged from the hospital and allowed to return home. But until then, my immune system was nonexistent and the doctor warned that a stray germ or sneeze could do me in.

Around the same time, the side effects of the chemo began to make themselves known. The lining of my throat began sloughing off, an excruciating side effect of the chemo called mucositis, which made it impossible to eat or drink or talk at anything louder than a whisper. "Are you ready to party?" Younique joked the first time she hooked me up to an intravenous morphine drip. Blessed be the excellent nurses with excellent senses of humor: They make everything better. But even with the morphine, the pain was too intense to swallow much of anything. In addition to the needle marks and bruises that now covered my arms, a spray of tiny purple dots the size of pinpricks appeared all over my chest and neck. Without platelets, the component of the blood that helps the body form clots, the capillaries closest to my skin had broken open, leaking blood to the surface. I avoided looking at myself in the mirror.

And then it finally happened: One morning, I woke up and discovered a mess of stray hairs on my pillow. By lunchtime, it was falling out in clumps, leaving pale patches all over my scalp. I ran my fingers compulsively over my skull, placing handfuls of my hair into little nest-like piles on the bedside table. Losing my hair was confirmation of what I knew but hadn't been able to fully accept yet and I spent the rest of the afternoon fighting back tears. That evening, Will helped me tug the rest out with his hands; it was like pulling weeds from damp soil. By bedtime, I was completely bald.

It had been more than four weeks since I'd entered the hospital, and I was waiting for my blood counts to recover from the chemo, but to my dismay they were showing no improvement. The doctors reassured me that there was no need to worry—at least, not yet—but of course, I did anyway. In the meantime, my body had become entirely reliant on transfusions. The blood of strangers coursed through my veins, bag after bag, day after day. Sometimes I tried to imagine who these donors were—a schoolteacher, a famous actor, a tarot card reader? I couldn't quite conjure them, but they were keeping me alive.

Being poked and palpated and locked in a room for days on end without a release date was maddening. The windows didn't open. The fluorescent bulbs scalded my eyes. My stomach hurt, my head hurt, my limbs hurt, everything hurt, even breathing. Each time I was stabbed with a needle or given a sponge bath, I wanted to hurl my IV pole at the wall. When I lost enough weight that I could slip off my electronic hospital bracelet, I began to fantasize about escaping. Central Park taunted me from my window. During a rainstorm, I felt a visceral longing to go outside and stand in the downpour—even if just for a minute. Finally, on a day when my pain had fleetingly retreated to a tolerable level, I hid my electronic bracelet under my pillow and when the nurses weren't looking, I ducked into the hallway and slipped into the elevator with my IV pole. I made it as far as the cafeteria on the ground floor. Then I froze. It was lunchtime, and people swarmed around me, brushing and bumping me. My anxiety mounted as I thought of all the germs in the air. I was having trouble breathing. What if I fell? What if I fainted? A few minutes later, I was back in my room. *Beep, beep,* my IV chirped. Strangely, I felt safe again.

If anyone could understand what I was living, it was the other patients, but I wasn't allowed to interact with them anymore, as the germ risk was too high. I missed their camaraderie and I tried to keep tabs on their progress through games of telephone facilitated by the nurses. Estelle had been discharged, and she was recuperating back home in Staten Island. Dennis's latest scans had lit up like the Milky Way, a constellation of new tumors in his lungs. He, too, would eventually need a bone marrow transplant. As for Yehya, he still walked by my room in the afternoons and, if no one was looking, he'd crack open the door, flash me a thumbs-up, and tell me Allah had my back.

I was still allowed visitors from the outside, but even that had become complicated. The people I'd played beer pong with in college had not reached out, and even though I was not surprised, I felt wounded by their silence. Instead, I tried to focus on those who did show up—my friend Mara, who came to see me nearly every day, and a cohort of old childhood pals, classmates, and colleagues, who stopped by with gifts. In the days after my diagnosis I'd welcomed their company, even craved it. But over time, I grew allergic to the looks of pity and the positivity pushers who tried to cheer me up with their get-well cards and their exhausting refrains of "stay strong" and "keep fighting." I began to feel angry at people's trivial complaints about a stressful day at the office or a broken toe that meant they couldn't go to the gym for a couple of weeks, and it was hard not to feel left out when my friends told me about a concert or a party they'd been to together.

Worse were the disaster tourists: those whom I didn't know well but who came out of the woodwork, showing up unannounced at my hospital room door with an overzealous desire to help or to bear witness to the medical carnival that my life had become. They would gape at my bald head, all misty-eyed, and I'd find myself having to console them. Or they'd bombard me with unsolicited medical advice, telling me about a great doctor they knew or a friend of a friend who'd cured their own cancer with things like essential oils, apricot kernels, coffee enemas, or a juice cleanse. I knew that most meant well and were doing the best they knew how, so I smiled and nodded, but I was silently fuming. As I got sicker, fewer and fewer came—and when they did, I began pretending to be asleep.

I wasn't entirely alone, despite my attempts to retreat from the world. Dr. Holland came to visit me nearly every day during his lunch break. He was gracious toward the nurses and the hospital staffers. Unlike some of the other attendings, who could be brusque and condescending, his bedside manner was unhurried and he always treated me with dignity, careful to make me feel like a person first and a patient second. After he was done examining me, he would sit in the recliner next to my bed, and we'd chat about everything from politics to art history and our favorite books.

Will, who was still unemployed, virtually lived in my hospital room, sleeping next to me every night on a too-short visitor's cot. My parents took the day shift, taking turns sitting by my bed and plying me with all of my favorite snacks in an attempt to get me to eat. Since entering the hospital, I had shrunk from a healthy size six to a double zero—the same size I'd been in the sixth grade—but I was often in too much pain to swallow, let alone choke down a forkful of mushroom risotto. I tried to perk up when they were around, but it was hard to stay awake for longer than a few minutes. My mother bought a poster of a Vermeer painting and hung it on the wall next to my bed. The painting showed a young woman playing the lute in a darkened room, her face turned to the window, her expression pensive and outward. "She reminds me of you," my mother said.

I knew how lucky I was to be surrounded by such love—many patients in the ward had no one to visit them at all—but even with my parents and Will by my side, I felt achingly isolated. My post-diagnosis euphoria and all my lofty plans had long since evaporated. I no longer had the energy to journal. My knitting needles and the half-completed scarf gathered dust. I never did read *War and Peace* or any of the other books on my bedside table. I was bored, nearly to death, but too exhausted to do anything about it.

One afternoon, after more than five weeks in the hospital, a team of doctors in baby-blue face masks appeared in my room. They loomed over my hospital bed, peering down at me. Eyes and ties. And white lab coats. "I'm afraid we have some bad news," a masked mouth said. "When you entered the hospital, you had thirty percent blasts in your bone marrow. Your latest biopsy results show that the number of blasts has more than doubled, to about seventy percent."

"Can you come back when my mom is here?" I whispered. I suddenly felt like a child.

Later, with my parents by my side, my medical team explained that I was going into bone marrow failure and that the standard treatments were not working for me. My father looked gutted. My mother seemed like she was about to break down, but when she caught me looking at her, she quickly blinked back her tears and rearranged her face into a more stoic expression. The doctors recommended I enroll in a phase II experimental clinical trial, meaning it was not yet known whether the new chemo drug combination was safe and effective, let alone better than the standard of care. At a time when everything already seemed so uncertain, I didn't want an experimental trial. I craved hard facts, statistics, and proof that my treatments were worth the havoc they had wreaked on my mental and physical health, and on the lives of my loved ones. As much as I was for scientific research, I had no desire to be a guinea pig. I wanted a cure.

"Wouldn't I be better off spending this time with you guys or smoking pot on some tropical island, or whatever it is you're supposed to do when you're dying?" I asked my parents. No one knew what to say. The doctors didn't have any answers for me either, but they kept insisting that the trial was my best option, and that the longer I waited, the fewer options I might have left. In the end, I agreed.

On the Fourth of July, the eve of my twenty-third birthday, I got special permission to leave the Bubble for a couple of minutes, the first time I'd stepped outside of my hospital room in nearly six weeks, with the exception of my aborted escape plan. I had heard a rumor that you could see the fireworks from the back corridor, by the elevators. After donning the mandatory protective armor, Will and I walked down the hallway, dragging my IV pole behind us. We stopped by Yehya's room to see if he wanted to join. He was too tired to get out of bed, but he had gifts waiting for me on the bedside table—a pink friendship bracelet and a wooden plaque painted in bright primary colors with the words I'M SUCH A BIG YOU FAN! that he'd asked his wife to procure from the hospital gift shop. Will helped me put on the bracelet and carried the plaque. Then we collected Dennis, and the three of us walked past the nurses' station and out of the ward.

When we arrived, a group of patients were already clustered in the back hall, peering out the windows. From behind the thick glass we could see only dimly, like goldfish peering out of a dirty aquarium. But if you angled your body down to the left and craned your neck to the right, you could catch glimpses of the fireworks in the distance. They were red and blue and gold; they exploded high into the sky, spraying color over the skyscrapers, but they were miles away and we couldn't hear their bursting from behind our soundproof barrier. The fireworks, the city, its inhabitants—the world—felt as far away as the moon. Meanwhile, the alarm on an old man's IV machine had gone off and it wouldn't shut up, the beeping enough to make anyone snap.

"Sorry to swear," I said, turning to Will and to Dennis, "but this is the most depressing fucking thing I have ever seen." My shoulders shook. At first, I thought I was going to cry, but then I burst out laughing. All of a sudden, everyone was laughing. Giggles and roars and oceanic tears at the absurdity of it all.

10

STOP-TIME

AFTER ALMOST TWO months in the Bubble, my doctors sent me home for a couple of weeks, to regain some strength before I began the clinical trial. My blast count was still terrifying—high enough that were it not for how weak I was, I would have started the new chemo drugs immediately. But the risk of the drugs killing me outweighed the risks of the blasts continuing to multiply in my marrow and blood. So, sicker than I'd ever been but off all treatment, I returned to Saratoga.

Stepping out onto the porch, I luxuriated in the movement of my legs, the in and out of my breath, the sun on my skin. Like an inmate released after a long sentence, I marveled at everything: a light rain misting my face; the sight of fireflies blinking in the garden at twilight; the smoky scent of barbecued ribs rising from our neighbor's grill over the hedge between the houses.

I tried to make the most of my newfound freedom. Whenever I was feeling well enough, Will would help me into the minivan, bundle me in blankets, and we'd go for long drives in the country-

side. If I had the energy, we'd go for a walk. Downtown Saratoga
was an eight-minute stroll from the house; twenty if you had leukemia. The annual horse-racing bonanza that draws bettors, tourists, and big-hat wearers each summer was in full swing. On every
street corner there were buskers playing music. The main drag,
Broadway, was crowded with a rowdy contingent of Harley motor-
cyclists, who parked their bikes in long rows along the street, and
die-hard gamblers, who eschewed the track for dive bars where
they could watch the races on television.

Being outdoors was a welcome change from the Bubble, but
with my lunar-bald head, lash-less eyes, disappearing eyebrows,
and face mask, I quickly became aware of the stares. Back in the
cancer ward, I'd looked like everyone else. Now everywhere I went,
I stood out. Cancer spoke for me before I could say the first word,
and rooms went quiet when I walked in. There were perks to this;
I got lots of free coffees and ice cream cones that summer, moist-
eyed cashiers saying, "Feel better, honey. This one's on the house."
But other times, the stares made me feel like a freak. One afternoon, as I stepped out of the bathroom at the public library, a little
girl pointed at me and screamed.

More often than not, I wasn't well enough to venture outside.
A bone-crushing exhaustion kept me leashed to the old leather
couch in the living room, with Will by my side. He had a knack for
transforming my bad days. "Movie day," he'd announce, as though
we were electing to spend the daylight hours inside. "You have a
big black hole in your knowledge of American pop culture, so I've
made us a curriculum. Today, we're tackling the late eighties. We'll
start with *Ferris Bueller's Day Off, The Breakfast Club,* and *Coming to America.* Then we'll break for lunch."

The caregiver's life is ultimately dictated by the cycle of decay
and demands of someone else's body. Will had moved into this
new role with an enthusiasm and a devotion that awed everyone.
Each morning, he helped my mother prepare homemade rice pud-
ding, the only thing I could stomach, and verbena tea infused with

fresh sprigs of mint, which was supposed to help with nausea, and then he would bring everything up to my room on a platter so I could eat in bed. He assisted my parents with chores around the house, and played basketball in the afternoons with my brother, who was home for the summer. He organized my pillbox, changed the dressing covering my catheter, and came with me to every single doctor's appointment. Will never complained, even when it meant missing out on parties or beach trips with friends. He reassured me again and again that there was nowhere else he'd rather be than by my side. I liked to think that if our situations were reversed, I would have had the patience and selflessness to care for him the way he did for me, but a part of me doubted that was true.

Will's folks visited that summer, traveling all the way from California to show us their support. It was my first time meeting them, and I wondered what they would think when they saw me in the flesh, all blanched and gray, with tubes protruding from my chest. I worried that a part of them would wish for a different kind of significant other for their only son. Someone like Will's ex, who had a full head of silky blond hair, a staff writer position at a prestigious magazine, and working ovaries—someone with prospects instead of a prognosis.

If his parents felt this way, they didn't show it. They pulled up to the house, all booming laughter and bear hugs. Within minutes, his father, Sean, a towering Irishman with a white mustache and twinkling blue eyes, pulled me aside. "My son is a better man since he met you," he told me. "I want to thank you for whatever it is you've done to him." His mother, Karen, a radiant blond hippie who wore linen dresses and colorful beaded jewelry, shared her son's knack for making everyone in his radius feel good. She told me over and over how beautiful and bold I looked with my bald head. "You should keep your hair short once you're better," she said.

Together, our families spent the weekend exploring Saratoga.

We strolled through the rose gardens of Yaddo, a famous artists' colony on the outskirts of town. We went to the racetrack and made two-dollar bets on the horses with the best names. (Somehow we lost every time.) In the evenings, we feasted in the backyard under the vine-covered lattice that my mother had decorated with string lights and paper lanterns. Our parents got along so well that it was hard to get a word in at dinner. Sean, a journalist and documentary filmmaker who had covered the war in Iraq, talked Middle East politics with my father, while our mothers bonded over their love of the arts. Will and I exchanged furtive winks and eye rolls across the table as our parents droned on.

On the last day of their visit, we all walked to the farmers market in town. The sun beat down on my wide-brimmed blue straw hat. I struggled to keep up as they wandered from stall to stall, sampling homemade blackberry preserves, olives, and cheese. Excusing myself, I wandered to a picnic table, where I took a seat in the shade of a tree. The twang of a fiddle and the shrieks of children chasing one another across the grass whirled around me, making me dizzy. I fanned myself with the hat, wishing I could teleport back to the quiet and cool of my bed.

When it was time for us to head home, I lagged behind, trying to conceal a limp. I didn't want to ruin what had otherwise been a perfect weekend, but by the time we reached the house, my limbs trembled and my sundress was soaked in sweat. I hugged Will's parents goodbye, promising to visit them in California when I was well enough, and then retreated into the house. "How are you feeling?" my parents asked when I hadn't budged from the couch for several hours.

"All good," I insisted, clenching my teeth. A dull, aching pain pulsed between my legs like a heartbeat. I was too embarrassed to explain its location—to say to my mother, or to my old-fashioned, bow-tie-wearing male doctor, or to anyone else, for that matter: *My hoo-ha hurts,* or some other anatomically vague description. I hoped the pain would go away on its own. But a few days later, I could no longer walk at all. As Will and my family sat down to dinner, I lay on the couch, my teeth chattering feverishly. When my mother took my temperature, the thermometer read 101. "That's it, we're going to the hospital," she ordered.

My mother drove, and Will sat next to me in the backseat, cradling my head in his lap, as we sped down the black highway. Every half hour or so Will checked my temperature, which continued to rise. My mother accelerated, her brow taut with worry. Three hours later, by the time we reached the Tappan Zee Bridge that crossed over the river toward Manhattan, she was going twenty miles above the speed limit and I had a fever of 104.

It was a Sunday night in the emergency room at Mount Sinai. The waiting area was packed, people pacing by the vending machines, some slumped half-asleep in plastic chairs or clutching bloodied appendages wrapped in gauze, mothers cradling wailing babies, diabetics hobbling on swollen feet. Everyone was waiting for the gatekeepers—the intake nurses and receptionists—to call their name. Triage, the process by which medical experts determine who gets seen first, can elicit survival-of-the-fittest impulses. Everyone feels their emergency should be the priority, and to have your needs, let alone your kid's needs, ranked among those of others can instill a sense of panic. Crowded emergency rooms do not bring out the best in people.

"My daughter has leukemia and a very high fever," my usually graceful mother snarled at the receptionist, forty-five minutes after we showed up. "She is severely immunocompromised and if you make her wait any longer you will have blood on your hands." Her threat worked, and for a brief moment, we felt victorious as a nurse came to collect us. But on the other side of the emergency room's swinging stainless steel doors, the chaos was even greater. Gurneys covered every square inch of the floor. Patients cried and moaned, some wailing for help. A woman in a wheelchair with a feral, unfocused gaze ranted at no one in particular, claiming that she had been poisoned by her co-workers.

There was nowhere to go, and barely any room for Will and my mother to stand. I remember looking at Will and thinking he seemed overwhelmed. My mother must have thought the same thing, and suggested he take a break if he needed one. "Yeah, I guess there's not much point in all three of us being here," Will said. "I might go meet a friend for a drink." A few minutes later he was gone.

I was placed in a bed an arm's length from a young man with matted dreadlocks. He lay motionless with his eyes closed, his soiled clothing making a sharp contrast against the fitted sheet of the gurney. A doctor whisked a curtain closed between us for privacy, but I could still hear every word of their conversation. Over the next few minutes, I learned the young man had AIDS and that he had a hemoglobin count of 3.0.

"Do you want a blood transfusion?" the doctor asked.

"No," the young man mumbled.

"Then you realize you're going to die, right?"

"Okay."

Not long after, a hospital worker came around to distribute sandwiches to the patients. The young man was too weak to hold his sandwich and it fell to the ground between our beds, lettuce and slices of pale deli meat splaying across the linoleum. "Is he all right? Someone needs to help him," I cried out to my mother. That's the last thing I remember before my eyes rolled back.

The next twelve hours unfolded in a series of feverish blackouts punctuated by brief pinpricks of fluorescent light.

Frame One: I woke up to a trio of doctors peering between my legs with flashlights. My face flushed with humiliation. I kept trying to push my knees together, but a gloved hand forced them apart. "Small cut in the inner labia," said a voice from behind a face mask. "Infection, possible sepsis," said another. "Let me get a look?" asked a third. The skin around the cut, they said, was necrotic.

Frame Two: "Where am I?" I asked, panicking. The steel mouth of an elevator yawned open onto a floor of the hospital I didn't recognize. I was wheeled into a small airless white cube of a room with hazy orange overheads. A nurse explained that I had been admitted to the geriatric unit. The hospital was at full capacity, and I would have to spend the night here until a room opened up in oncology. This struck me as hilarious—indeed, my body felt twenty-three going on eighty—but I didn't have the energy to explain to anyone why I was cackling, as if someone had delivered a particularly excellent joke.

Frame Three: *I'm so cold, I'm so cold, I'm so cold,* I repeated to my mother, but with each blanket she layered over me, the colder I felt. Nothing could warm me. My teeth clacked violently and I began to shiver uncontrollably. "Can we get a doctor in here?" someone shouted. Later, I'd learn I was having something called a "neutropenic fever," meaning I had almost no infection-fighting cells left to do battle for me.

Frame Four: My temperature shot up and up and up until the thermometer read 105.8. When I tried to speak, my words came out in garbled, foreign tongues. My body, seized by rigors, shook and soiled itself. Will appeared in the doorway just as a nurse was attempting to wedge a bedpan beneath my naked flanks. "Tell him to wait outside," I moaned to my mother, suddenly coherent, as I covered my face with my hands.

Frame Five: My usually smiling oncologist, Dr. Holland, was not smiling when he showed up. "Call your husband and tell him to come to the hospital," I overheard him tell my mother. It was the middle of the night, my father was back home in Saratoga, a three-and-a-half-hour drive away. "Can it wait until morning?" my mother said. "I don't want to frighten him." Dr. Holland put his

hand on her shoulder and looked her square in the eye. "Anne.
Call your husband. This could go either way."

When I came to the next day, my eyes rolled wildly around the
room as I tried to piece together where I was and what had happened. My parents sat next to my bed, looking several decades
older. A nurse leaned over me, handing me a paper cup with an
oxycodone pill. Within minutes, I was retching into the plastic
basin by the hospital bed. The drugs and the realization that I was
alive crashed into me like a freight train, my relief soaring across
the boundary into euphoria.

The rooms were bigger and nicer in the geriatric unit than
those in oncology. I liked it here, except for the nurse with the
bottle-blond hair who talked too much. "I used to work in oncology," she said as she lodged the silver tip of a thermometer under
my tongue. "I remember a girl named Joanie. She was a sweet girl,
around your age. Every time she came in with a new infection, I
wanted to cry. When she died, it was just too sad. Just looking at
you makes me sad, makes me think of Joanie. So now I work here,
in geriatrics."

Illness had made me good at separating my scripts. There were
the words I kept in my head—*please stop talking, don't you see we
are already so scared*—and the words I actually spoke out loud:
"Joanie was fortunate to have you as a nurse."

That night, Will arrived to take over for my parents. He stretched
out awkwardly in the reclining chair next to my bed, covering himself with a thin cotton blanket. The geriatric unit was all out of
visitor's cots. Tonight, like so many other nights, he would sacrifice comfort for closeness.

"I think we should get married," I said, out of nowhere, the oxy
making my tongue a little too limber. I worried that if we waited,
we'd never get the chance.

"I'm all in," Will replied without missing a beat.

We stayed up late into the night excitedly ironing out the logistics, the invite list and which of my musician friends we would ask to perform. I called my two closest friends from college, Lizzie and Mara, who jumped into action, offering their help. Lizzie and her mother would take Will ring shopping in the diamond district; Mara volunteered her family's home as the venue for the ceremony. It would be a small wedding, a simple autumn shindig in the backyard, with a handful of our closest friends and family. Barring more emergency hospitalizations, we hoped to have it soon—ideally in the next few weeks.

A few days later, a room opened up in oncology and I was transferred upstairs. Just three months earlier, the oncology unit had felt like a foreign country; now, perversely, I felt at home among the chorus of beeping IV monitors and the bald-headed patients. I belonged. When I saw Younique we greeted each other like girlfriends reuniting after a long spell apart. "Why hello, Miss Suleika! I heard you were back. How are you and that fine man of yours?"

"Getting married," I gushed.

I asked how my friends from the floor were faring. Younique sat on the edge of my bed, smoothing a blanket over me with gentle hands. Yehya was gone—"No, not back to Algeria," she corrected me. He had died in the room with the beautiful park views, his wife by his side. As for Dennis, he'd been making progress toward transplant until, one afternoon, his organs started to shut down in swift succession. Despite the doctors' best efforts, they hadn't been able to resuscitate him. No one ever came to claim his body.

Younique rubbed my back as I tried to process the news. All I could think was, *I'm next.*

11

STUCK

I'VE ALWAYS KEPT a journal. The bookcase in my childhood bedroom is filled with dozens of colorful notebooks, each one detailing a new chapter in my life. The pages read like conversations with myself, expressed in thick, swooping pen strokes: fever-dream visions for the future, lies about late-night adventures I never took but wished I had, thinly veiled autobiographical short stories driven by aspirational female protagonists, bad poetry, and lists, always lists—of dos, don'ts, and dreams. My twelve-year-old self had different types of conversations from the ones I had at sixteen, or at twenty. But they all shared something in common: They were looking ahead.

With mortality in the balance, one of life's most delicious activities when you're young—imagining your future—had become a frightening, despair-inducing exercise. The future had once seemed infinite with possibility. Now it was shrouded in doom, a dark space ahead filled only with the promise of more poisonous treatments and terrifying unknowns. Thinking about the past stirred a nostalgia I preferred not to dwell on, a painful reminder of all I had lost, was losing: my friends; my youth; my fertility; my hair; the "milestone necklace" my parents had given me on my first day of chemo, which had gone missing somewhere in transit between the hospital and home; my mind, as the chemo made me cloudy and slow; my faith that I would ever make it to transplant.

Living with a life-threatening illness turned me into a second-class citizen in the land of time. My days were a slow emergency, my life dwindling to four white walls, a hospital bed, and fluorescent lights, my body punctured by tubes and wires tethering me to various monitors and my IV pole. The world outside my window seemed farther and farther away, my field of vision shrinking to a tiny pinpoint. Time was a waiting room—waiting for doctors, waiting for blood transfusions and test results, waiting for better days. I tried to focus on the preciousness of the present: the moments when I was well enough to walk around the oncology unit with my parents, the sound of Will's voice as he read out loud to me each night before bed, the weekends when my brother came to visit from college—all of us together now, while it was still possible. But try as I might, I couldn't help but feel an incipient grief and guilt as my thoughts turned, inevitably, to what would happen to Will and my family if I didn't survive.

The infection had set me back by a couple of weeks, but the clinical trial was slated to begin the moment my doctors deemed me strong enough. I was one of 135 patients in the United States who were enrolled in the trial. The first nine days of each month I would receive a combination of two potent chemo drugs, azacitidine and vorinostat, and then I'd have roughly two weeks off to recover, before beginning the next cycle. The trial would be outpatient, meaning that when I wasn't in the city for doctors' appointments or hospitalized for complications, I would get to stay at home in Saratoga. The whole process would take six months—that is, if everything went as planned.

As the leaves on the old maple tree in my parents' backyard turned a crisp, burnt orange, an uneasiness began to shadow my long hermetic days with Will. He had been my constant companion since my diagnosis and it was his intention to remain so throughout the clinical trial. Selfishly, I loved getting to spend so much time with him. Even though I was bedridden, bald, occasionally incontinent, and living with my parents, the very fact of having a boyfriend gave me a sense of normalcy, of still being young, wanted, even beautiful. But some part of me knew the situation wasn't sustainable. The land of the sick was no place for anyone to live 24/7; I would never have wished it upon my worst enemy. I knew that if I wanted our relationship to last, I would need to encourage Will to start living his life again.

"Let's find you a job," I said gently to him one afternoon. We'd just finished a fifth consecutive game of Scrabble.

He sighed. "I know, I know, I've been thinking about that, too. I really could use the income right now. But I don't want you to feel like you're alone in this."

"I'm not getting better, at least not anytime soon," I said. He acknowledged that he couldn't put his life on hold indefinitely.

At first, Will searched for jobs that were close to my parents' house, but other than bartending or waiting tables in downtown Saratoga, there wasn't much to choose from. We widened the search radius and when I noticed an opening for an assistant editor position at a big news outlet in Manhattan, I pushed Will to apply. He was hesitant. Saratoga was a three-and-a-half-hour drive away—too far to commute back and forth every day. If he got the job, it would mean being apart during the workweek. When Will expressed concerns about the distance, especially when the trial was coming up and my health was so tenuous, I brushed them off. I wanted him to be happy, but a part of me was living vicariously through him, too. It was a job I would have loved to have had in the alternate reality where my body wasn't trying to destroy me. So I threw myself into helping him—revising his cover letter, practicing with him for the interview, and finding him a free place to live in a friend's apartment during the week in the event that he got the job. When the phone rang to say the position was his, I hugged him with all the force left in my frail bird bones. "Things are about to get better for us," I said, and I meant it.

Not long after, on a brisk autumn morning, we headed to the Saratoga train station, where Will climbed aboard the Ethan Allen Express to begin his first week of work. As he turned to look back at me, I beamed a high-watt smile, then waved at him enthusiastically until the doors closed. Standing on the platform, I watched the wheels rumble along the tracks, heard the train as it whistled around the bend and disappeared. Alone, I felt my excitement dampen, then darken.

Back at my parents' house, I walked up the stairs to my room, locked the door, and lay flat on my bed, facedown. I remained there immobile for a while, holding my breath. Then I howled into my pillow—a deep, blood-vessel-popping howl of frustration and envy directed at Will, at my friends, at everyone else who was out there starting jobs, taking trips, discovering new things—all unencumbered by illness. That everyone's lives were starting while mine was over before it had begun seemed unspeakably unfair. When I'd run out of air, lungs burning, I stood up and walked across my room to the small wooden desk pushed up against the windows and flipped open my journal.

The world is moving forward and I am stuck, I wrote.

With Will gone during the week, it was tempting to let myself stew in self-pity, so I began searching for something productive to do with my time. First, I decided to enroll in a creative writing course at Skidmore, the college down the road from our house where my father was a professor in the French department and my brother was finishing his senior year. But I only ever made it to the first day of class. By then, the clinical trial was under way, and within two weeks I was admitted back to the hospital with another neutropenic fever. The sores in my mouth multiplied and grew so painful that when I was discharged, my medical team prescribed me a fentanyl patch, an opioid a hundred times more potent than morphine.

My days were spent in bed, propped semi-upright by pillows. Until my cancer siege, I had always prided myself on being ambitious. The detritus of past achievements that filled my childhood bedroom—ribbons, trophies, awards, and diplomas—now mocked me. Determined to keep searching for something to do with myself, I decided to start studying for the GRE with the idea that I could apply to graduate school. I spent the next few weeks brushing up on algebra, taking practice tests, and researching PhD programs in International Relations and Near Eastern Studies. I was hospitalized again before I could sign up for the exam—this time for an infection caused by the catheter in my chest, which was surgically removed and replaced by a new one—but as soon as I was back home, I registered to take the GRE later that week, before another complication could hijack the plan. On the morning of the exam, my mother made me a special breakfast of "brain-boosting foods": scrambled eggs, with a side of sautéed kale and porridge with ground flaxseeds and blueberries. I did my best to take a couple of bites, even though I had no appetite. As she drove me to the testing center in Albany, I napped in the backseat, trying to conserve energy. When we arrived, a surly receptionist informed me that I wasn't allowed to wear the knit hat covering my bald head during the exam. My mother explained that I was undergoing chemotherapy, but the receptionist was unmoved. "It's the rules."

Shivering in the temperature-controlled air, my bald head gleaming under the bright lights, I was determined to finish that damn test. It took me the full three hours and forty-five minutes to do it. By the end, I was delirious, my eyelids drooping with exhaustion and my teeth clacking feverishly, but I finished. When I received my results a few weeks later they were mediocre, but I was undeterred. Over the next month, I threw myself into applying to a handful of PhD programs across the country, soliciting recommendation letters from former professors, drafting the necessary admission essays, and filling out scholarship forms. When I finally hit Submit on my applications, I expected to feel victorious but deep down I knew my efforts had been in vain. Even if I got into graduate school, there was no way I'd be well enough to attend.

I stopped writing in my journal after that. I grew resigned to the idea that, for the time being, I had one central preoccupation: ongoingness. The clinical trial was proving harder on my body than anyone could have predicted. The toxicity of the drugs was so intense that at the end of each cycle I was rushed to the emergency room and admitted to the hospital for multi-week stays, battling more neutropenic fevers and life-threatening complications ranging from colitis to sepsis. My mouth was so blistered with sores that even with the fentanyl patch and a cocktail of supplementary drugs, I was in perpetual pain. I began keeping a bottle of liquid morphine on my bedside table and whenever the pain roused me in the middle of the night, I would take a couple of sips until I could fall back asleep. I started to wonder if the side effects of the clinical trial and the painkillers I was prescribed would kill me before the leukemia did. I often thought about quitting the trial altogether. If it weren't for the pleas of Will and my parents, I think I would have.

During one of my many hospitalizations that fall, I shared my wedding plans with my medical team. I expected them to be excited at my good news, but their reactions were more concerned than celebratory. Within the hour, a social worker appeared at my hospital room door, asking to speak to my parents and me. "The goal is to get you to bone marrow transplant," she said. "As I'm sure you know, this is an expensive procedure—a transplant can cost more than a million dollars. Luckily, you're on your father's insurance, which will cover the majority of the cost, but getting married could jeopardize your eligibility to stay on his policy. We just don't think it's worth the risk. At least, not until you're out of the woods."

I glared at the social worker. She was young and pretty with long, lovely strawberry-blond hair streaming past her shoulders. On a slender, perfectly manicured finger, she wore a giant diamond engagement ring. I knew she was just the messenger, and I knew she was right, but I couldn't help but hate her for it. The wedding was postponed, joining the countless other plans and goals and projects that had been relegated to purgatory until further notice. No one spoke of it again.

A kind of sundering was taking place within me: There was the good-natured patient, young and spunky and cheerful, who raged courageously against her disease, determined to make the best of her terrible circumstances, and this new version, envious, short-fused, sleeping sixteen hours a day and rarely ever leaving her room. On Sunday nights, when Will packed his bags, preparing to leave Saratoga for the workweek, I wanted to put on a happy, supportive face. I tried. But as the weeks passed and I got sicker, it grew harder. It was unfair of me to resent him for going—not least because I was the one who had convinced him to take the job—but an anger unlike any I'd experienced before was building inside me, contained for now, but threatening to consume everything around me. Will, the social worker, everyone else who was out there participating in the world—they weren't the enemy, the disease was. I knew that, but with each day, each dream deferred, it got harder and harder to tell the difference.

12

CLINICAL TRIAL BLUES

MY PARENTS BECAME convinced that I was depressed that winter. I had taken to pressing the button on my IV pole that delivered a bolus of morphine straight to my veins as often as possible. I looked forward to the smoky chemical twilight, a welcome respite from my mind's incessant chatter. I talked less and less, drawing inward. Sometimes, out of frustration and anger, I lashed out, only to retreat even deeper. *L'appel du vide* beckoned; my moods sank into dark ruts from which I no longer knew how to lift myself.

When I wasn't sleeping or feeling seasick from the clinical trial drugs, I was busy setting the world record for the number of *Grey's Anatomy* episodes watched consecutively. When one episode ended, without even thinking, I would begin the next, desperate for a distraction from my rapidly deteriorating mental and physical state. There was something strangely soothing about TV medical dramas—gruesome wounds gushing torrents of fake blood, patients coding on surgical tables only to be rescued by gorgeous doctors, fleets of ambulances screeching into the hospital parking lot following yet another epic, citywide tragedy. Flooding my brain with these images numbed me to my own medical drama. It also gave me an exciting narrative and some steamy plot twists to project onto the packs of young residents I saw roaming the halls. One day, while at the hospital, I asked one of the residents if her life bore any resemblance to those of the doctors on the show. "Everyone is significantly less attractive," she said. "But we have just as much sex."

My favorite thing to watch when I wasn't bingeing on *Grey's* was a movie called *A Little Bit of Heaven*. In it, Kate Hudson plays a free-spirited young woman who gets diagnosed with colon cancer—or "ass cancer," as she calls it—and falls in love with her handsome oncologist. Spoiler alert: She dies at the end, but there's a joyous funeral with pink umbrellas, fluttering streamers, champagne, and a second line parade. By all accounts, including mine, the movie is terrible, but it was one of the only depictions of cancer in youth that I had come across and it made me feel a little less isolated. Each time I watched it—and I did so dozens of times—I would cry inconsolably for hours, which was a relief, because I'd been finding it difficult to feel much of anything as of late. It allowed me to face the one topic my friends and family refused to discuss, even though it was on everyone's mind: the possibility that I could die, and soon.

In light of all this, it's unsurprising that my parents were concerned—and that they were vocal about it. "Why don't you go to a cancer support group, or reach out to some of your old Saratoga friends?" they said. "Take a break from TV, get out of the house for a bit, do something fun. Wouldn't that be nice?"

I had no interest in attending a support group, but made an effort to reconnect with some childhood friends for the same reason I allowed myself to be poisoned over and over again with experimental pharmaceutical drugs that had yet to be proven effective and safe: I didn't want my parents to worry any more than they already did. I reached out to Molly, whom I'd known since pre-school, and who lived a few towns over, where she worked at a local bee farm. We talked on the phone one day and made a plan to hang out at the mall, the only meeting place for suburban young people with a serious shortage of things to do. When the day arrived, I pulled a rumpled blouse and a pair of black jeans from my suitcase, which stood, still unpacked from Paris, in a corner of my room. The clothes hung off my skeletal body, but I had nothing else to wear. I had long ago traded in civilian clothes for the patient's uniform: comfy sweats, robes, pajamas, and slippers. My feet had grown so slender and bony that I had to borrow a pair of my mom's boots, a half size smaller than mine. I covered my bald head with a hot-pink wig, adjusting it in the mirror. Peering into my makeup bag for the first time in months, I contemplated drawing on some eyebrows, but I was interrupted by my mother's energetic ringing of the cowbell.

"Don't forget that I need to give you your injections before you go!" she hollered from the bottom of the stairs.

My body tensed when she appeared in the doorway of my room holding two syringes. The clinical trial nurses had trained her to administer the chemo injections. This had seemed like a good idea, allowing me extra time at home before I was inevitably admitted to the hospital for another neutropenic fever, but I'd quickly come to dread the ritual, a metallic tang of fear coating my tongue at the sight of the needles. I knew how fortunate I was to have a mother who cared for me with such dedication and devotion. Since my diagnosis, taking care of me had become her main focus. I tried to remind myself that some people, like my friend Dennis, had no one to care for them at all. But in the moment, it was difficult to locate my gratitude.

My mother sat on the edge of my bed and got to work cleaning my upper arm in gentle, concentric circles with towelettes of rubbing alcohol. "I'm sorry, I'm sorry, I'm sorry," she said preemptively. With every day, the injections had become more torturous.

Even though my mother was careful to alternate arms, by the end of each trial cycle, the skin around the needle sites peeled off in sheets. Beneath the needle sites, rock-hard cystic lumps had formed, the lightest touch making me cry out in pain. As my mother slid the first needle into the muscle, I grimaced, then yelped. By the time she finished the second, I couldn't look her in the eye. The logical mind tries to remind itself that sometimes you must suffer in order to feel better. But the body has its own memory: It remembers who hurt it. On an irrational level, I felt wronged by those whom I saw as having "poisoned" me (people in lab coats, phlebotomists, my mother) and by those who encouraged me to think positively about it (friends, Hallmark cards, the "cancer books" section of Barnes & Noble). Finding the silver lining felt like part of the punishment.

Much later, my mother would share with me her diary from that winter: *I call my friend Catherine to cancel my tea time with her tomorrow morning. I want to say: "Catherine, how is this happening to us, to Suleika?" And instead I say this and I say that, I ask about her son and her husband. It makes me feel better and wounded at the same time, because what I have to tell is about transfusions and fatigue and reality. The tears are in my heart but they never come out. Only when Suleika doesn't speak to me do I lose all strength. Communication, love, laughter, her presence—that's what makes this bearable, what allows us to keep going like Ulysses.*

Maybe if I had read this then, it would have made a difference—though in all truthfulness, I doubt it. Suffering can make you selfish, turn you cruel. It can make you feel like there is nothing but you and your anger, the crackle of exam table paper beneath bruised limbs, the way your heart pounds into your mouth when the doctor enters the room with the latest biopsy results. But I wasn't the only one whose life had been interrupted by illness; my loved ones all faced a rupture that was similar in kind, if not in degree. That I wasn't the only one in the room meant I was one of the lucky ones, I knew.

My mother went straight to bed, as she often did after the injections, and my father drove me to the mall. I had never gotten my driver's license, but even if I had, in my condition I wouldn't have been allowed behind a wheel. One of the side effects of being in cancer treatment and on a mother lode of painkillers was impaired motor skills and cognitive ability; another was helicopter parents who watched everything I did, hovering close at all times in case my body decided to call it quits.

"Why don't I park so that I can accompany you inside?" my father asked as he pulled up to the mall's entrance.

"I've got it covered, Pops," I replied, trying to conceal my frustration. I hated how, ever since my diagnosis, everyone, especially my parents, treated me like a baby.

I walked around the food court looking for Molly. When I couldn't find her, I took a seat in front of the Burger King, trying to steady the squelching sensation in my stomach by taking deep breaths. I chalked this up to nerves. The last time Molly and I had hung out was in junior high. An incident one hot summer day involving a bottle of vodka, tacos, and multiple hours spent sunbathing had ended with Molly projectile vomiting and her mother screaming at me that I was a "terrible influence." We hadn't been allowed to hang out again. After college, Molly had moved back home to take care of her mother, who now had Alzheimer's. As soon as Molly had heard the news of my diagnosis, she sent me a heartfelt note, asking if I wanted to get together. I was resistant, not wanting to take her up on an offer that I thought had surely been made out of pity, but as I waited for her, I realized I no longer cared. Now that I was out in the world, I was thrilled to have weekday plans with someone other than my parents or the cast of *Grey's Anatomy*.

Molly finally arrived, half an hour late. She looked the same but was taller, with wild blond hair that tumbled down her back and black combat boots that made her already long legs look even longer. She apologized for making me wait, then said, "I made a

quick stop on my way over. Thought it might help with the chemo."
She winked and handed me a small cloth pouch fragrant with
weed.

We made small talk as we walked to the cinema and bought
tickets to the next showing, then settled into the overstuffed seats
of the theater. I tried to focus on the movie, but the smell of popcorn and stale sweat made my stomach squelch harder. Just as I
felt the familiar panic rising up my esophagus, it hit me: In my
rush to get ready, I had forgotten to take my antinausea medication before the chemo. I sprinted from my seat, trying to reach the
bathroom in time, but I only made it as far as the trash can next to
the concession stand. I retched and I retched and I retched, my
body shuddering violently. A group of teenage girls standing in
line looked on. "Ew," said one. "Bitch is *wasted*," snickered another. I ignored them. It wasn't the first time I'd publicly disgorged
the contents of my stomach since starting the clinical trial and it
wouldn't be the last. I was growing accustomed to losing my dignity in front of strangers.

When I was done, I returned to my seat, as though nothing had
happened. I wasn't ready to go home yet, even though I felt trem-
bly and nauseated. For just one night, I wanted to pretend like I
was a normal young person doing normal young person things. I
sat there with my eyes closed, trying to steady my stomach, until
the credits rolled across the screen.

Afterward, Molly drove me home. When we pulled up to my
house, the street was dark except for a pale light burning downstairs, illuminating the floor-to-ceiling red bookshelves of the
study. My father was sitting at his desk, bent over a stack of papers, reading something. *Probably medical stuff*, I thought. Nego-
tiating with the insurance company and decoding medical jargon
had become a full-time job.

"*Bonne nuit*," I said to my father, poking my head through the
doorway of his study before retreating upstairs to my room.

"How was it?"

"So much fun," I said. I didn't want to upset him with the truth.

My father looked exhausted. He had dark circles under his eyes and his face was sallow and sagging in new places. I felt an impulse to hug him, to tell him I loved him, but we didn't have that kind of relationship.

"Molly gave me this," I said, plopping the weed-filled pouch onto his desk. "You look like you could use it more than me."

13

THE HUNDRED-DAY PROJECT

"**YOU NEED TO** find a hobby, something you can do that's *within* your physical limitations," said the therapist my parents had forced me to start seeing. Her words seem obvious now, but at the time, I experienced them as an epiphany. The wedding, the creative writing class, the GRE, the applications to graduate school, the trip to the mall with Molly—these were all things that would have made sense in the context of my former life. I needed to find something I could do from home or a hospital bed. I needed not only to accept my limitations—the exhaustion and nausea, the brain fog and constant hospitalizations—but to figure out a way to make something useful from my pain.

"I hear baking can be quite soothing," the therapist suggested. She lost me there. People were often making such suggestions to me. Hospital volunteers offered a variety of activities to break up the day—knitting and beading, making vision boards and dream catchers. Friends sent me jigsaw puzzles, "adult" coloring books, and board games. But none of these activities felt very *me*. I'm *sick,* I wanted to say—not retired or in preschool.

In the end, though, I agreed to try something we called the Hundred-Day Project. I don't know who came up with it first, but the idea was that my family, Will, and I would each carve out a few minutes to work on a creative project every day for the next hundred days. The project was meant to be a way of organizing our lives around one small act of imagination; with time, it became much more.

For Will's Hundred-Day Project, he decided to send me daily video dispatches from the outside on everything from the weather to the quality of the pizza in the hospital cafeteria. "Today, I'm reporting live from Central Park," he said in one. "I'd like to introduce you to my favorite hot dog vendor. Rafiki, say 'what up' to Suleika." I watched and rewatched the videos whenever I felt lonely. I worried sometimes that the distance between us was becoming unbridgeable, but the videos helped me feel connected to him, to the world outside my window.

As for my mother, she decided to paint one small handmade ceramic tile each morning. At the end of the project, she assembled the tiles into a big multicolored mosaic that she hung on the wall of my bedroom. "Suleika's Shield," she called it, telling me it had protective powers. She tried to hide her pain in the art, but I wondered if the images, mostly of birds in distress—falling, upside down, beaks open in despair—reflected her own state of mind. *Le coeur qui saigne,* the heart that bleeds, one tile noted.

For my father's project, he wrote down 101 childhood memories that he printed and bound into a little book that he gave to me on Christmas morning. It was my first real glimpse into his past. He wrote about his family's annual spring outings to visit the shrine of the patron saint Sidi Gnaw, in the Matmata caves of Tunisia. He wrote about my great-great-grandmother Oumi 'Ouisha, the town healer, who would send my father to fetch the herbs and desert plants she kept under her bed as she murmured incantations into her patients' ears. He wrote about the shock he felt as a boy when he first visited the "French beach" on the other side of town, where colonial expats lounged in bikinis and Speedos. "Our women, when they bathed in the sea, which occurred once a year during *Awossu,* waded knee-deep into the water fully clothed. We called them 'floating tents.'"

One entry haunted me long after I read it. It was the story of my father's younger sister, Gmar, the one "with the beautiful face." I had never heard of her—I had never heard anyone in my extended family even utter her name, which means "moon" in Arabic. As I read on, I understood why. Gmar had spent most of her short life in bed, enfeebled by a mysterious disease, until one blazing summer morning when "she expired," as my father put it. He was four years old when Gmar died, but he could still hear his mother's wails echoing through the house. He never dared ask her what had ailed Gmar for fear of stirring painful memories. To my knowledge, there was no history of cancer in my father's family, but finishing the story, I couldn't help wondering if Gmar and I shared a diagnosis. In a strange way, it was comforting to think that I wasn't the only one.

As for my Hundred-Day Project, I decided to return to what I had always leaned on in difficult times: keeping a journal. I promised myself that, no matter how sick or exhausted I felt, I would try to jot something down every day, even if it was nothing more than a sentence.

People often respond to the news of tragedy with "words fail," but words did not fail me that day, or the next, or thereafter—they poured out of me, first cautiously, then exuberantly, my mind awakening as if from a long slumber, thoughts tumbling out faster than my pen could keep up. This was different from any kind of writing I'd done in the past. There was nothing future-looking about it. Each sentence was grounded in the now. I'd always imagined myself as the kind of writer who would help other people tell their stories, but increasingly I found myself gravitating toward the first person. Illness had turned my gaze inward.

As a patient, you are constantly asked to investigate the body, to report on yourself, and to narrate your findings: *How are you feeling? What is your pain on a scale of one to ten? Any new symptoms? Do you feel ready to go home?* I understood now why so many writers and artists, while in the thick of illness, became memoirists. It provided a sense of control, a way to reshape your circumstances on your own terms, in your own words. "That is what literature offers—a language powerful enough to say how it is," Jeanette Winterson wrote. "It isn't a hiding place. It is a finding place."

There were days, of course, when I was too tired to write much, but keeping a journal rekindled my love of words, and that inspired me to begin reading seriously again. My mother had given me a hardbound copy of *The Diary of Frida Kahlo,* and I pored over it. I was moved when I learned that—at an age not much younger than I was when leukemia struck—Kahlo had been a premedical student in Mexico City. One day, while riding home from school, her bus collided with a streetcar. She suffered fractures of the clavicle, ribs, spine, elbow, pelvis, and leg. Her right foot was crushed, and her left shoulder was dislocated. She was pierced by the streetcar's iron handrail, which entered her left hip and exited through her pelvic floor. The injuries left her bedridden for months.

Before the accident, Kahlo had dreamed of becoming a doctor. Afterward, she had to abandon those plans, but all that time stuck convalescing at home pushed her to uncover a new passion. "I never thought of painting until 1926, when I was in bed on account of an automobile accident," she said. "I was bored as hell in bed with a plaster cast . . . so I decided to do something. I [stole] from my father some oil paints, and my mother ordered for me a special easel because I couldn't sit [up], and I started to paint."

Kahlo transformed her confinement into a place incandescent with metaphor and meaning. Using a small lap easel and a mirror hung overhead in the canopy of her bed so that she could see her reflection, she began painting the self-portraits that would make her one of the most famous artists of all time. But the plaster corset she wore to brace her injured spine—the body itself—served as Kahlo's first canvas, a canvas she returned to again and again. Throughout her life, she had dozens of corsets, objects of both torture and beauty, imprisonment and inspiration, that would define the trajectory of her existence and her career. She adorned each one, covering the plaster with scraps of fabric and images of monkeys, brightly plumed birds, tigers, and streetcars. Sometimes she painted her scars, even her tears. "I paint myself because I am so often alone," she said. "I am my own muse, I am the subject I know best. The subject I want to know better."

Kahlo's surgeries and convalescences, infatuations and heartbreaks, lived on in her paintings after she died, and she eventually gained a near-mythical status as a patron saint of misfits and sufferers. Could these masterpieces ever have been painted by someone who was well? I wondered. Could they have been created by someone who hadn't been forced to confront the terrible fragility of the human body? I wasn't sure.

I was no Frida Kahlo, of course, so it was still difficult for me to imagine how I might creatively engage with my own misfortune. But her story had ignited something inside of me. I began to research the long lineage of bedridden artists and writers who alchemized their suffering into creative grist: Henri Matisse, while recovering from intestinal cancer, had worked on his design of the Chapel of the Rosary in Venice by pretending the ceiling of his apartment was the chapel, and attaching a paintbrush to a long pole, which allowed him to work from bed. Marcel Proust had lived lying down as a result of the severe asthma and depression that had plagued him since childhood, and penned his seven-volume epic, *In Search of Lost Time,* from a narrow brass bed in his bedroom, which was lined with cork to buffer him from the sounds of the outside world. Roald Dahl believed his chronic pain had been the creative springboard for his career as a writer: "I doubt I would have written a line, or would have had the ability to write a line, unless some minor tragedy had sort of twisted my mind out of the normal rut," he wrote in a letter to a friend. In all of these cases, it was the very fact of being physically limited, of life being foreclosed in other ways, that seemed to heighten imagination and embolden productivity. As Kahlo wrote, "Feet, what do I need you for when I have wings to fly?"

I decided to reimagine my survival as a creative act. If the chemo sores in my mouth made it too painful to talk, I would find new ways to communicate. As long as I was stuck in bed, my imagination would become the vessel that allowed me to travel beyond the confines of my room. If my body had grown so depleted that I now had only three functional hours each day, I would clarify my priorities and make the most of how I spent the time I had.

With this in mind, I reorganized my bedroom so that everything I needed was within arm's reach: a small night table littered with pens, notebooks, and paper; a bookshelf filled with my favorite novels and volumes of poetry; a wooden board that I placed atop my knees as a desk. I wrote when I was home, and I wrote each day that I found myself back in the hospital. I wrote until the anger and envy and pain bled dry—until I could no longer hear the persistent beeping of monitors, the hiss of respirators, the alarms that constantly went off. I had no way of predicting all the places the Hundred-Day Project would take me, but what I knew, for now, was that I was starting to find my power.

14

TANGO TO TRANSPLANT

NEARLY A YEAR earlier, shortly after my diagnosis, I'd called my brother, Adam, on Skype while he was studying abroad in Argentina. I had to tell him that I'd just been diagnosed with leukemia and that—no pressure—he was my only shot at a cure. At first he thought I was playing a twisted prank on him. "This isn't funny," he said. "I'm serious," I said. "I wish I were joking." My parents and I had kept him mostly in the dark about my condition, hoping to shield him from worry, and as it dawned on him that this was not, in fact, a joke, his face fell. Without question, he took a leave from his study abroad program and, a few days later, boarded a plane to New York to undergo the necessary tests.

The results showed that Adam was a match—a perfect match, a ten out of ten on the donor scale—and we celebrated, overjoyed by this bit of good news. We were in such good spirits that we could, in fact, find humor in the circumstances. Soon after, my brother christened me with a new nickname. "*Salut,* Suleikemia," he'd say each morning. But then, the reality of what was to come began to sink in—that suddenly everyone in our family was leaning on my brother. Adam insisted he was glad to be able to do something to help, but it was an enormous amount of pressure to be under. By the time the clinical trial got under way, he was a senior in college, and while his friends were applying to jobs and partying away the final months of the school year, he was shuttling from campus to the city for appointments with my transplant team. On top of that, my parents were terrified that he might do something that would put his health at risk, so they began badgering him not to drink or smoke or stay out too late. One night during dinner my mother made a comment about his sugar intake and Adam lost it. "What is this? Some fucked-up version of *My Sister's Keeper*?" he shouted before storming out of the room. In the months that followed, he struggled to keep up with his studies and reduced his course load. He started taking medication for anxiety and, when he came home on weekends, I could hear him tossing and turning in his room next door.

All of this added to the guilt that had been my steady, secret companion since my diagnosis. I felt guilty about the financial distress I was causing my family. The piles of medical bills and copays. The lost income. When I got sick, my mother had turned her focus from painting to being my full-time caregiver, and my father often missed class because of my medical emergencies and was beginning to wonder if he should take the next semester off. I felt guilty whenever I spiked a fever in the middle of the night, knowing one of them would need to drive me the three and a half hours to the city, streaking down the highway to reach the emergency room in time. I felt guilty after my father returned from his long afternoon walks in the woods, his face puffy. I felt guilty when Will turned down a promotion at work. He didn't say it was because of me, but I knew it was. He was already pushing it with his boss, always asking to work remotely so that he could keep me company in the hospital, exhaustion ringing his eyes from all those nights sleeping on a cot, rest made impossible by the ceaseless beeping of monitors. I felt guilty about my brother who didn't talk much about his feelings but who confessed one night to my mother that, as my donor, he felt responsible for the outcome of my bone marrow transplant. I felt guilty about what my illness had done to my family, the pain and stress I was causing everyone, the amount of "space" my body took up with its problems. It was impossible not to feel like a burden.

After each round of the clinical trial, the doctors performed a bone marrow biopsy, checking for lurking leukemic blasts, the ten-inch needle notching a new scar on my lower back. For the most part, the results showed progress, but it was slow. "Just a few more rounds," Dr. Holland would say at the end of a treatment cycle. For months it went on like this, until finally—endless biopsies and near-fatal complications, and months of hospitalizations later—we hit a magic number. While the clinical trial hadn't completely eradicated my leukemia, the number of blasts in my marrow had dipped under 5 percent, a safe enough level for me to move on to what we all hoped would be the final phase: transplant.

Dr. Holland did his best to prepare me and my family for what was to come. He told us that I would spend about eight weeks in the transplant unit. During my first week, I would undergo an intensive regimen of chemo designed to wipe out my marrow and immune system so that my body could receive my new marrow. I was familiar with the nausea and vomiting that accompanied chemo, but Dr. Holland warned us that the treatment would be far more aggressive than any I'd received. My body would have to ward off fevers and mucositis without any white blood cells to protect me. I would likely need a feeding tube, and I would be connected to a 24/7 morphine drip.

The week before the transplant, my brother would be given injections to stimulate the production of stem cells, the primitive marrow cells that mature into red blood cells, white blood cells, and platelets. Forty-eight hours before the transplant, my brother would enter the hospital so that his stem cells could be harvested. For roughly nine hours, he would sit in a hospital room, with a needle in one arm, hooked up to a machine that would filter the stem cells from his blood plasma through a process known as apheresis. Once a sufficient amount of stem cells had been collected into IV bags, they would be injected into the central line implanted into my chest. My fate lay in those stem cells, in their ability to move through my blood and to find their way into my marrow, where they would hopefully begin to grow and proliferate. The two weeks after transplant would be the most difficult as we waited to see if the transplant had worked—if the stem cells successfully engrafted into my marrow. Assuming the transplant succeeded, the donor cells would slowly replenish my marrow and create a new immune system. Once my blood counts stabilized, and once I no longer needed transfusions, I would be discharged. I would have to find a place to live close to the hospital, so that I could come in for daily checkups. The recovery period would take several months, until my new immune system was strong enough for me to go outside without a protective face mask and gloves.

Among cancer patients, a bone marrow transplant is considered a rebirth, a second birthday—but only if it works. The transplant itself is dangerous. One of the biggest potential complications is graft-versus-host disease (GVHD), which occurs when the graft (the donor's cells) does not recognize the host (the patient's cells) as derived from the same self. Immune cells relentlessly attack what is foreign—that's how the body eradicates infections—but in the case of GVHD, the patient becomes the target. The first symptoms, which typically appear within the first hundred days after transplant, can be as mild as a rash but they can also be far more serious, ravaging the lungs, liver, eyes, and gastrointestinal tract. Even if the transplant worked—even if I did not develop GVHD— I would still be extremely susceptible to infections and a raft of other complications, including heart failure and organ damage.

My doctors told me and my parents that I had about a 35 percent chance of long-term survival. *Thirty-five percent*. When I heard it, the number whooshed and rattled through my bones. And even if I did survive "long term," the possible side effects, which ironically included a high risk of new cancers in the future, were also terrifying. I felt as though I was walking around with a loaded gun pressed against my temple. A medical game of Russian roulette.

Before my diagnosis, the phrase "carpe diem" had always struck me as a cliché, something you heard in that sappy Robin Williams movie or in college graduation speeches. Now, as the transplant neared, each day felt like a carpe diem countdown. I felt a need to make the most out of every single thing I did. Every day, every hour, was invaluable and not to be wasted. Time stalked me like prey. I wasn't the only one to feel this way. For the first time ever, my mother arranged to have a family portrait taken by a professional photographer. Will and my closest friends threw me a party that felt part "godspeed," part "goodbye." And my father started saying *"je t'aime"* to me each night before I went to bed. I had always felt fiercely loved by my father, but it was the first time in my life I could remember hearing him say it out loud.

I was moved by all these gestures, but I was a bit frightened, too. When you are facing the possibility of imminent death, people treat you differently: Their gaze lingers, recording each mole, tracing the shape of your lips, noting the exact shade of your eyes, as if they are painting a portrait of you to hang in memory's gallery. They take dozens of pictures and videos of you on their phones, trying to freeze-frame time, to bottle the sound of your laugh, to immortalize meaningful moments that can later be revisited in a memory cloud. All of this attention can feel like you are being memorialized while you are still alive.

But what scared me more than the transplant, more than the debilitating side effects that came with it, more than the possibility of death itself, was the thought of being remembered as someone else's sad story of unmet potential. My most significant accomplishments as an adult had been fetching coffees and making photocopies as a paralegal, and doing my best to fight a disease I'd never wanted in the first place. I hadn't done anything I was proud of yet. I had spent my twenty-three years on this planet preparing for a life: pulling all-nighters so that I could get the grades to receive a scholarship to a good college and, one day, have a career of my choosing; learning to cook for the dinner parties I told myself I'd throw one day; saving up my paychecks to be able to go on a long trip somewhere; talking about all the writing I wanted to do without ever actually working up the courage to put any of my writing out into the world. I knew it was likely too late for most of these things, but I was determined to seize the days I had left. Facing my mortality had stripped away any concerns about being cool, and it did not feel embarrassing or too earnest to say that I hoped to make a difference. I wanted, in my own way, however small, to contribute something to the world. To leave more than I took.

After almost one year spent in isolation, shuttling between the hospital and my parents' house in Saratoga, I was done hiding. "It is always what is under pressure in us, especially under pressure of concealment—that explodes in poetry," Adrienne Rich wrote. I wanted to understand what had happened to me, to excavate its meaning on my own terms. I wanted the last word to be mine.

So, I decided to start a blog.

The idea was to create some kind of platform for a population of people who are too often misunderstood and overlooked: young adults with cancer. I didn't know what this would look like yet but I began to document my time in bed and in the hospital. With my parents' support and Will's help, I got to work. I enlisted a photographer friend from high school to take pictures; I got ahold of a cheap video camera and spent hours shooting and editing little videos; I pored over YouTube tutorials, teaching myself how to build a basic website; and finally, in preparation for the blog's big launch, I drafted my first posts, culling from some of the writing I'd done for my Hundred-Day Project.

I took myself and my new blog very seriously. "I'm on a deadline," I would tell the nurses when they came around to check on me or to adjust my medications. Of course, these deadlines were entirely self-imposed, but it felt so good to have a job to do—to have a purpose other than just being a patient.

When the blog went live in early 2012, my expectations were low. I was pretty sure that my readership would consist of only Will and my parents, possibly my grandmother. But to my surprise my first post began to be shared, not only by relatives but also by friends, classmates, and even my college journalism professor, who wrote to say that he was impressed, and that he planned to send it around to some colleagues. When I woke up the next day, I discovered that *The Huffington Post* had featured my first blog entry, titled "Good Afternoon, You Have Cancer," on the home page: "Today, as I prepare for a bone marrow transplant, I've learned that my biggest challenge might not be physical," I had written. "It is enduring the boredom, despair, and isolation of being sick and confined to a bed for an indeterminate length of time." Within hours, my humble website had thousands of views. I posted a second entry, this one more tongue-in-cheek, called "10 Things Not to Say to a Cancer Patient," with an etiquette guide for the friends of those living with life-threatening illness. Soon, I was getting letters from people who were not tied to me by blood or acquaintance—perfect strangers from all over the map.

One of the first letters I received was from a young man by the nickname of Lil' GQ, who wanted me to know that my story had touched, as he put it, *a death row convict heart*. But the real reason he was writing was because, in a strange way, he related to my predicament. *I know that our situations are different,* he wrote in flowery cursive, *but the threat of death lurks in both of our shadows.* While Lil' GQ had never been sick, he, too, was stuck in limbo, awaiting the news of his fate.

As I lay in my hospital bed in New York City reading and re-reading his letter, it was surreal to imagine Lil' GQ in his cell fifteen hundred miles away in Texas. There was so much I wanted to ask him, so much I wanted to know. I wondered if he, like me, ever plotted his escape. I wanted to know if his fear of death was the same as my fear of death. Or if it felt different to await your execution, not at the hands of a disease, but at those of uniformed guards sanctioned by the law. I was hungry for more details about Lil' GQ's past—about how he'd ended up on death row. I was curious about what he did to pass the time. How do you wake up each day, how do you continue on when the future spells uncertainty, or worse, certain doom?

I made a couple of stabs at a response, but I couldn't write him back. The blog consumed what little energy I had. Too weak to sit at a desk, I wrote from bed, propped up by a mountain of pillows. The chemo had made my thoughts slow and sticky, and I worked haltingly, in ten-minute bursts staggered throughout each day. For extra energy, I slurped iced cappuccinos. The syrupy slush cooled my inflamed mouth and the caffeine helped keep me somewhat lucid. When I was too sick to type, I dictated out loud to Will, who sat at the foot of my bed, tapping away on my laptop, giving me feedback and encouragement. It was arduous, exhausting, satisfying work.

Two weeks later, as I waited to get a final biopsy before beginning the transplant process, an email arrived. It was from an editor at *The New York Times* who had read my blog and wanted to know if I'd like to write an essay for the paper. The thought of a byline sent a charge of excitement through my body, and I suddenly wanted to jump up and down and do cartwheels in my hospital room. I wrote an email back and included my phone number, and to my surprise the editor called me right away.

"Interested?" the editor asked.

"Possibly," I bluffed.

I had never been published in a real newspaper before. I had never worked with an editor. I *had* been rejected from the creative writing program freshman year of college, and, other than the two journalism classes I'd taken as electives, I had never formally studied writing at all. But during those many hours of writing in my journal and dreaming up my blog, an idea kept percolating in my mind, growing more insistent, until I could think of nothing else. I ached to find language for the mysterious happenings in my bones, for those endless months of lying in bed, forced into a state of solitary reflection, for all those humiliations and flirtations with the fatal, for the experience of witnessing the serial deaths of fellow patients, as well as parts of myself. In truth, I had no idea what I was doing and I certainly didn't know if I was well enough to pull it off. But I knew I had almost nothing to lose. Cancer made me brazen.

"What I'd really love to write is a weekly column about the experience of illness in youth," I said.

Pitching a column to *The New York Times* as an unpublished twenty-three-year-old was more than a little presumptuous. I understood that instead of funneling what little energy I had into writing, I should have been resting my body, preparing for transplant, and spending time with my family. I should have paused to ask myself how sharing the most difficult moments of my life in real time might impact my health, my future, my loved ones. But there I was, pacing around the room on my cellphone in my blue cotton gown as I made my case to the editor, explaining how I planned to harness all that had happened to me since my diagnosis, and to translate these experiences into thousand-word weekly installments. Maybe the column could be accompanied by a video series, I proposed, explaining that I knew firsthand how hard it could be to read when ill and that I wanted the project to be as inclusive as possible.

"Okay," the editor replied. "We'll try the column for a couple of installments and see how it goes. I'll connect you to one of our filmmakers on staff, so that you can discuss the possibility of a video series. Let me know when you finish a draft of the first column."

I hung up the phone and burst into tears.

"What's wrong?" my mother asked, alarmed.

"I think I just got a job."

"Write," instructs Annie Dillard, "as if you were dying." We are all terminal patients on this earth—the mystery is not "if" but "when" death appears in the plotline. With my transplant date looming, her words rang loudly. My mortality shadowed each breath, each step that I took, more present now than it had ever been. A manic energy hummed through me. I worked around the clock for a month to draft thirteen columns before I entered the transplant unit, fueled by the knowledge that it was going to be a long time before I was well enough to write or walk or do much of anything else again. What would you write about if you knew you might die soon? Bent over my laptop in bed, I traveled to where the silence was in my life. I wrote about my infertility and how no one had warned me of it. About learning to navigate our absurd healthcare system. About what it meant to fall in love while falling sick, and how we talk—or don't talk—about dying. I wrote about guilt. I also wrote a will in case I fell on the wrong side of the transplant odds. To this day, I've never been more prolific. Death can be a great motivator.

On March 29, 2012, my column and an accompanying video series—called "Life, Interrupted"—was scheduled to make its debut. Just a few days after that I would receive the bone marrow transplant. The confluence of these impending milestones was dizzying: a dream and a nightmare dancing the tango.

15

ON OPPOSITE ENDS
OF A TELESCOPE

ON MY FIRST night in the bone marrow transplant unit, I lay in my hospital bed, eyes wide, under a halo of hanging IV bags. My fear was alive. I could smell its wet fur in the room and feel the chuffing of its breath, hot on my skin. Folding back the blankets, I stepped out of bed and over the thick vine of tubes and wires that connected me to various machines. Dropping to my hands and knees as my late pal Yehya had done—careful not to bang my head—I pressed my forehead to the cool linoleum. With a father who had been raised Muslim and a mother who had been raised Catholic, I'd grown up with a mishmash of beliefs and traditions. When we were with our Swiss side of the family, we celebrated Easter and went to Mass; when we were with our Tunisian family, we fasted during Ramadan and slaughtered a lamb on Eid; and when we were in the United States, we retained a fairly secular existence, with the exception of Christmas. While I'd always had a great interest in religion, I'd never truly practiced one myself. I didn't know how to pray, or to whom, but this much was clear to me: I needed all the help I could get.

What was it that I was asking for, exactly? How many other desperate folks had tried bargaining with a higher power in this same hospital room? I was beginning to feel dizzy, my emaciated legs trembling under the weight of my body. Heaving myself up, I grabbed a glow-in-the-dark pen a friend had gifted me and made my way to the wall. I had no poetry, no eloquent manifesto to impart. Just one simple, animal desire: *Let me live*, I scrawled in tiny letters—part prayer, part plea.

The intensity of the moment was heightened by my new surroundings. After researching the top transplant units, I had decided to transfer my care from Mount Sinai to Memorial Sloan Kettering Cancer Center, which was considered the best transplant unit in the city, if not the country. Still, I fretted over the decision. Shopping for bone marrow transplant units had been a bit like visiting colleges—other than the glossy brochures and swift meet and greets, only time would tell if I'd made the right choice. In Sloan Kettering's transplant unit, with all of its beeping monitors, futuristic equipment, and unfamiliar faces in surgical gowns and masks, I felt as if I'd boarded an alien spaceship. I missed Dr. Holland and my medical team—our inside jokes, their nerdy brilliance and blazing compassion. Over the last year, my doctors and nurses had come to feel like extended family. "Promise you'll come back to visit me once you're better," Younique had told me when we said goodbye.

The last week had been full of goodbyes. I spent my few final days before entering the transplant unit in Saratoga. I had packed my red suitcase in preparation for the eight-week-long hospital stay, adding, at the last minute, Sleepy, the stuffed dog I'd cherished as a kid. I hadn't been able to sleep on the eve of my departure, so I got up at five o'clock and wandered the house. I took a last look at my childhood bedroom, bidding goodbye to those pink walls, bookshelves, and old favorite posters. Running a hand over the wooden nape of my bass, I said goodbye to it, too. I said goodbye to the dining room table, where we'd shared countless meals as a family through the years, and to the frozen flower beds of my mother's garden. Will and my parents came down for breakfast and loaded our bags into the car. I felt a sinking sadness as the minivan pulled away from the house, wondering if I would ever return. For the person facing death, mourning begins in the present tense, in a series of private, preemptive goodbyes that take place long before the body's last breath.

In the transplant unit, I was surrounded by people who were concerned, first and foremost, with what I had—not necessarily who I was. Doctors and nurses in masks stood over my hospital bed, peering down at me, discussing me as if I weren't in the room. They gave the Patient a hospital gown. The Patient was talked at, looked at, probed, prodded, and whispered about. They had a singular goal—to cure the Patient so she could go back to being herself. In all this lay a strange irony: It had only been a year since my diagnosis, but I could hardly remember what being myself was like.

Over the course of the next week, my immune system was blasted with twenty infusions of heavy-duty chemotherapy—more chemo than I'd had in the year since my diagnosis. During all this, I kept my hospital room neat. I had always liked organizing and arranging, but my tidiness became almost obsessive-compulsive as I stacked my books, pills, and water bottles into ruler-straight rows on my bedside table. I refused to don a hospital gown, wearing instead my own pajamas, robe, and sheepskin slippers. Each morning I rose from bed and moved to the fold-out couch in my hospital room that I made up with fresh sheets and blankets. I had brought a portable speaker from home, and as I revised my *New York Times* columns and responded to emails, I blasted James Brown or Bach to drone out the sounds of the hospital. I worked furiously, eager to get as much as I could done before the side effects of the chemo intensified. Inevitably they did, so as I typed, I kept a yellow vomit bucket tucked under one arm.

On the morning of the transplant—Day Zero, as it's called—my parents and Will arrived at my hospital room wearing yellow surgical gowns and blue face masks. My brother followed, with his usual greeting. "*Salut,* Suleikemia," he said, leaning over to give me a fist bump through our latex gloves. I laughed, then replied, "Hope I never have to hear that again." A few minutes later, half a dozen doctors and nurses filed into the room, and what levity had filled the air dissipated.

Given all the anticipation, the actual procedure was somewhat anticlimactic. Everyone stood solemnly in two rows, flanking my bed like a regiment of soldiers, watching as my brother's stem cells dripped from a hanging IV bag. I felt calm as the last drops emptied into my veins, perhaps because I was not there, not really. I closed my eyes and began imagining myself across an ocean, on another continent, sitting in a café with Will in Paris, then strolling down the streets of Tunis. My body was strong, my hair long again.

Within minutes it was over, and everyone filed back out of the room to let me rest.

The hardest part, my medical team warned me, were the days and weeks ahead, as I waited for Adam's cells to engraft in my marrow. I was put back on "isolation" status. Precautions in the transplant unit were far more extreme than anything I'd experienced at Mount Sinai. A specialized vent in my room filtered out any impurities in the air. All of my food was nuked beyond recognition to kill off any potential germs. Anyone who entered my room had to wash their hands and to dress up in the equivalent of a hazmat suit—plastic gloves, a surgical gown, a face mask, and booties over their shoes. A kiss, a handshake, fresh fruits and vegetables, the common cold or a paper cut—these were all things that could kill me until my immune system began to work again. Even flowers were forbidden, though this seemed presumptuous to announce to friends and relatives, so bouquet deliveries gathered, unopened, outside my door.

The goal was to reach Day 100, or "Examination Day," the first major benchmark for evaluating a patient's recovery from the transplant. I tried to keep track of time from my bed, where I spent the days and nights lying at a forty-five-degree angle to prevent my lungs from filling up with fluid, but the hours melted together. My IV machine hung over my bed like an awning, carrying my daily intake of fluids, immunosuppressants, antinausea medications, three different kinds of antibiotics, and a round-the-clock morphine drip. The ceiling vent emitted the hiss of cold air, a constant, anxiety-inducing audio track.

I spent nearly two weeks this way, without any major incident. Then, in the early hours of Day 14, someone began to scream, a deep, steady wail, so loud it woke me up. The room was dark. An alarm was sounding. Tubes were wrapped around me like snakes. My chest was slick. I felt something wet spurting from below my collarbone, dribbling down my sides. A moment later, the door swung open and a nurse's face appeared over me. She squeezed my shoulder and it was only then that I realized the scream was coming from me. "Holy shit," she blurted, as she peered down at me in horror. I'd been having a nightmare: dozens of insects scurrying over me and gnawing at my skin. In a drugged panic, I'd ripped my catheter clean out of my chest.

There's a tipping point, a special kind of claustrophobia reserved for long hospitalizations, that sets in around week two of being locked in a room. Time starts to elongate; space falls apart. You stare at the ceiling for so many hours that you begin to see shapes and patterns, entire universes appearing in the cracks and crevices of the popcorn plaster. The walls begin to close in around you. When the pitter-patter of rain against the window wakes you from a medicated haze, you yearn for it, like nothing you've yearned for before—to be outdoors, to feel the rain drizzling down the back of your neck, to tilt your head up and taste the sky on your tongue. You try to open the windows, though you know full well that they are sealed shut. Your desperation begins to border on madness.

Most people don't know what it's like to live this way, locked in a tiny white room with no release date in sight, unless perhaps they've been incarcerated. While in the transplant unit I was often reminded of Lil' GQ, the death row inmate who had written to me a few weeks earlier. I wondered what he did to pass all that time in solitary confinement. I wondered how—if—he'd been able to maintain his sanity. Inspired in part by him, I began drafting a column in which I reflected on what I termed my "incanceration":

To a cancer patient, the lexicon of the prisoner seems to scream out from everywhere. Your movement is monitored. Decisions as basic as what and when to eat require pre-approval from a higher order. Not to mention that chemo-therapy feels like a semilethal punishment. The medical staff plays the judge. At any moment, your doctor can issue a sen-tence: probation, house arrest, extended time in "jail" and, for some, even death row. I've never had to appear in court, but I imagine the adrenaline pumps the way it does before a doctor reads your biopsy results.

Lil' GQ wasn't the only stranger whose words kept me com-pany during those long, delirious days in the transplant unit. Each morning, I checked my in-box to find it filled with dozens of notes from readers of "Life, Interrupted." Though I wasn't allowed to leave my hospital room, writing had given me a portal through which I could travel across time, space, continents.

I heard from all kinds of people, many of whom had been sick themselves. I heard from a teenage girl in Florida named Unique, who was undergoing treatment for liver cancer and sent me a message composed largely of emojis. I heard from a retired art historian in Ohio named Howard, who'd lived with a mysterious, chronic autoimmune condition for most of his life. *You are a young woman, I am an old man. You are looking ahead, I am looking back. It is likely that we have only our mortality in common,* he wrote. *Meaning is not found in the material realm— dinner, jazz, cocktails, conversation or whatever. Meaning is what's left when everything else is stripped away.* I heard from many who had never been sick a day in their life, but who related to the broader notion of having their life "interrupted." From the wife of a senator in the Midwest who was struggling with infertility. From a young man with bipolar disorder who had recently become homeless and was living out of his car in Boston. From Katherine, a high school teacher in California, who was mourning the death of her son.

I should have felt lonelier in the transplant unit than ever before, but these strangers and their stories quickly became my conduits to the outside world. I relished the letters I received, though I rarely had the energy to respond. When I did, my first priority was to write back to the young adults with cancer—they were my people, after all. One was Johnny, a nineteen-year-old boy from Michigan who was also being treated at Sloan Kettering for leukemia. He'd read my column and sent me a message on Twitter, and I replied right away. It was the first time I'd had the opportunity to talk with a young person who shared my diagnosis. Both of us were on "isolation" status, sequestered in our respective Bubbles on different floors of the same hospital, and we were forbidden from meeting face-to-face. We chatted online instead, our conversations drifting from the silly to the serious, often in the span of one long run-on sentence. We were both bombed out of our minds on morphine, which leveled any expectation of punctuation or spelling or grammar—a relief.

JOHNNY: What's your fav thing on the hospital menu?
ME: The QUESADILLAS.
JOHNNY: YES, had a quesadilla yesterday and was in heaven.
ME: Are u inpatient?
JOHNNY: Just got moved to the pediatric floor . . . I got the middle bed and the other guy has to walk past me to use the bathroom plus the view is totally not as good
JOHNNY: how are you feeling post bmt [bone marrow transplant]
ME: grumpy & irritated. the nurses come in to weigh me everyday at 5 am.
JOHNNY: I cant wait to feel life cancer free.
ME: same. do you know any spells to speed up time?

My heart ached for Johnny. Our shared experience was brutal, but between us existed a weird sort of beauty: There we were, two complete strangers, arms extending from our screens, wrapping each other in an intimate embrace.

Nearly three weeks after my transplant—or Day Plus 20, as the doctors and nurses referred to it—Will stood with his back to me, looking out the window of my hospital room, describing the morning scene to me as I lay in bed. Fractals of sunshine across the East River. The lip of a bridge poking out over blackened tenement buildings. Yellow taxis jerking down York Avenue like Monopoly pieces. Tiny hustlers in suits commuting to work. I wanted to join him, but I was too tired to get up and drag my IV pole the five feet to where he stood. I knew he'd be on his way to the office in a few minutes, but the drugs were making my eyelids heavy. When I woke up next, he was already gone.

Such sleep was a kind of refuge, a numbing to the side effects of the transplant. What little hair on my body that had grown back during the clinical trial was falling out again, leaving my skin raw and silky, almost larval. My weight had plummeted and my already skeletal torso shrank, but my cheeks had grown round and swollen from all the steroids and liquids being pumped into my system. *Moon face,* cancer patients call this. Shrunken and stretched in all the wrong places, broken blood vessels blooming like watercolor paint across the surface of my skin, I felt hideous—less moon face, more monster.

My immune system was completely wiped out. I was waiting for Adam's healthy stem cells to engraft, but it was taking longer than expected. Adam was finishing his last few weeks of college and he should have been focusing on finals and parties and graduation. But, like my parents and everyone who entered this sterile Bubble, he concealed his worry behind a mask.

Later that afternoon, I woke up to the sound of my parents' voices. As I twisted my head to say hello to them, I felt something inside my throat rip and detach like Velcro. I lurched forward, my mouth filling with blood, as I heaved up a hideous mass of flesh into the plastic bucket next to my bed.

"What happened?" my parents cried out in alarm, calling for the nurse.

"Your daughter just vomited up the lining of her esophagus," the nurse explained in a business-as-usual voice, calmly surveying the mess.

The chemo was burning away the mucous membranes that lined my mouth, throat, and gastrointestinal tract, which made it impossible to talk or eat anything other than ice chips. Hour after hour I vomited chunks of charred flesh into the bucket next to my bed. The pain and antinausea drugs provided some relief, but I spent much of my waking hours pretending to be a statue, trying to sit still in the hope that it might soothe my roiling stomach. When the doctors arrived, encircling my bed in a protective ring of yellow medical gowns, they hooked me up to a feeding tube, a direct line to a bag of greenish-yellow liquid that looked like Mountain Dew.

That evening, Will returned. He had skipped a work dinner to spend some time with me. I wanted to ask him all about his day. Did he do anything interesting? Did he have lunch in the park? Any office gossip? But we were interrupted by the nurse, who was hanging a new bag of medication. It would make me drowsy soon. Will offered to read to me, or to set up the Scrabble board, even if I was only up for a few turns. I couldn't remember the last time we'd played.

Will's schedule was full with his job and the basketball and soccer leagues he'd joined the week before I entered the transplant unit. On most nights, by the time he got to the hospital, I was already fast asleep. I knew he needed an outlet to cope with the stress of our situation—all caregivers do—but I couldn't understand why he was so busy all of a sudden. Increasingly, it felt as if we were peering at each other through the opposite ends of a telescope.

My teeth chattered as Will draped me in a heated blanket. He poured me some water in a Dixie cup. I wet my tongue and let the cold liquid eddy around my mouth—a momentary tonic for my swollen cheeks—before I spat it out. I didn't want to resent the hand holding the water jug. It was my body I was at war with. There was so much we needed to talk about, but I suddenly felt overwhelmed by a deep exhaustion. My eyelids felt heavy again. Will sat next to my bed. As I drifted off, we held hands through blue latex gloves.

16

HOPE LODGE

ROLLING OUT OF the hospital onto York Avenue in a wheelchair, I lifted my face up to the sun, letting it warm my sallow skin. It was a balmy May afternoon, but I was swaddled in a wool hat and a ski jacket, and my teeth, as usual, were chattering. The wheelchair clogged the busy sidewalk outside the hospital's main entrance, as I waited while my mother and Will hailed a taxi. Pedestrians stepped aside, inadvertent spectators to our little procession. My feet touched the sidewalk briefly as I got into the waiting cab.

It had been a little more than a month since I'd undergone the transplant. The doctors had told me that though my immune system was still nonexistent, preliminary tests showed that Adam's cells were finally beginning to engraft in my bone marrow. I was showing signs of progress: In the last few days I had transitioned from a feeding tube to being able to keep down a couple of saltine crackers, I was able to walk around—slowly—but without assistance for the most part, and my blood counts were creeping in the right direction. It would be several more weeks before we knew if the transplant had worked—Day 100 still loomed ahead—but for now, I was focused on a smaller victory: discharge.

The doctors were sending me to the Hope Lodge, a kind of halfway house for cancer patients in Midtown Manhattan, where I would live for the next three months. It was a gray concrete building with sixty rooms down the street from a Jack's 99-Cent Store and one block from Penn Station. For the foreseeable future, I would need to wear gloves and a mask everywhere I went. *No subways, no public places, no germs,* my doctors cautioned. I rolled from the taxi to the entrance, the sidewalk crowded with pedestrians. I pulled my face mask tighter over my mouth.

I was grateful that a place like the Hope Lodge existed, and grateful for the generosity of the strangers who had raised the money to open it, but in an ideal world, I wouldn't have had to live there at all. In an ideal world, I would've had my own place. I would have moved into my mother's first apartment in the East Village, which she had held on to for all those years, renting it until recently to long-term tenants. But my immune system was still too fragile to live in a ground-floor apartment of a prewar building right next to the dumpsters. More than that, it was too small for me to live there with both Will and my mother. It had become clear soon after my transplant that being a caregiver to a recent transplant patient was a round-the-clock job, one that my mother and Will planned to share. So we'd decided that I would stay at the Hope Lodge and that they could use the apartment as needed, as a sort of caregiver outpost. It was the best plan we could come up with given the circumstances.

It fell through the moment we arrived at the Hope Lodge. Inside, a receptionist greeted us and handed over a room key and a packet of information. Then Will and my mother began following me into the elevator to go upstairs to the room, only to have the receptionist call after us to say that only one caregiver at a time was allowed to accompany a patient on the residential floors—no exceptions. We tried to push back, saying that such rigid protocols didn't take into account the demands and the unpredictability of illness. But the rules were the rules, and it became clear that my hope for how Will and my mother would share caregiving duties—fluidly and in tandem, like a family—wasn't possible. There would be no spontaneity, no room for the two of them to support me together or to support each other. I would have to constantly choose between one and the other.

I was torn. I needed the kind of help you could only really ask for from a parent—but I felt like Will and I were drifting, and I didn't want to be apart. Since day one of my diagnosis, my greatest fear other than dying had been losing him, and now that I was sicker than ever, my instinct was to hold him close. So I suggested that Will live with me at the Hope Lodge, and my mother visit during the day while he was at work. At the time, it seemed like a good compromise.

The room Will and I shared at the Hope Lodge was a dingy setup—two twin beds, motel furnishings, and a brownish carpet, with a dearth of natural light. Down the hall was a communal kitchen where we'd bump into other caregivers and patients and have to stop for chitchat like "Just coming from the hospital?" or "How's the old brain tumor?" The atmosphere in the building was weighted down by sadness. Everyone who lived here had left behind a real life somewhere else.

The Hope Lodge staff worked hard to lift the mood. Downstairs, on the sixth floor, there was a living room with a fireplace and a spacious outdoor terrace where patients could sit and visit with friends and family. Classes were offered in the lounge on topics like Zen meditation and neutropenic-friendly cooking classes, and several times a week volunteers put on special events—concerts, comedy shows, and dinners donated by local restaurants. There was even a weekly "teatime" hosted by a gaggle of Manhattan ladies. Every Wednesday afternoon, they descended on the lounge dressed in Chanel pantsuits, tottering around on six-inch stilettos as they arranged platters of cakes and pastries. These women were well intentioned, I'm sure, but I couldn't stand how they spoke to us patients in loud, slow sentences, their voices dripping with condescension, as though we weren't just sick, but somehow didn't speak English. I quickly came to despise teatime. I didn't want their charity or their pity. I didn't want to be anyone's good deed of the week.

My post-transplant routine consisted mainly of sleeping eighteen hours a day. When I wasn't asleep, I lay in bed with my eyes closed, too exhausted to sit up, to talk, or to read. The only exception, strangely, was *Fifty Shades of Grey*. I inhaled the entire trilogy in one weekend. It was so beyond the pale, so different from my reality in every way, that it felt like science fiction. It was also the only thing engrossingly, comically terrible enough to distract me from the overpowering nausea.

"Classic would you rather," I said to Will one morning. "Acute myeloid leukemia or read *Fifty Shades*?"

"Leukemia," he said, without hesitation.

Will was fixing me breakfast, as he did each morning, though I rarely ate more than a bite. Then he'd pass me off to my mother before heading to work. The most dreaded part of my day was the daily trek from the Hope Lodge to the hospital, where I received blood transfusions, hydration, magnesium, and other nutrients that the chemo had wiped out. I was so nauseated all the time that I rarely completed the twenty-minute taxi ride across Midtown without getting sick. Once, during a particularly violent bout of backseat vomiting, a taxi driver thought I was drunk, and kicked my mother and me out of the cab. Before I could explain, he'd ditched us on the curb and driven away.

Less than a week after I moved into the Hope Lodge, I was invited to be interviewed about the column on NPR's *Talk of the Nation*.

It was a big day: my first real outing since leaving the hospital. After finishing up my IV infusions, my mother and I took a taxi to the NPR office across from Bryant Park. I had never been interviewed by anyone before, and I was buzzing with excitement.

I still couldn't quite comprehend why, but since the column's launch, I'd received all kinds of interview requests. Readers had begun walking up to me in the hospital's waiting room, a few even approaching me on the sidewalks of Manhattan, to tell me how much they loved the column and that they were rooting for me. This attention was flattering, more than a little overwhelming, and at times it left me feeling a bit uneasy. Cancer had turned me into an unwitting poster child.

Not everyone shared in the excitement. The column had rapidly become a source of tension with Will. He worried about the toll it took on my health and complained that I was pouring what little energy I had into work. He wasn't wrong; it was true that I could feel my ambition bumping up against the limitations of my body. My brain, flooded with toxins from all the drugs that had been pumped into my system, felt broken. Once able to remember vast amounts of useless information in great detail, from the color of my third-grade teacher's blouse on the first day of school to entire passages of my favorite books, I now struggled to recall the names of my closest friends or even my own cellphone number. Before the transplant, writing had been a refuge for me; now it most often resulted in frustration and tears. But I was determined to do what I could while I could, even if that meant pushing my body beyond the boundaries of what was prudent.

The evening before the NPR interview, I'd come down with a low-grade fever and spent all night under the covers shivering, a gnarly sounding cough raking through my lungs every couple of minutes. Will and my mother both begged me to reschedule, but I refused. I didn't know how long such opportunities would be available to me, or if I'd be well enough to do them again. I would

do the interview and there was nothing anyone could say to talk
me out of it.

By the time I'd settled into the recording booth at the NPR office and the sound check was completed, I was exhausted. My
hands were unsteady as I sipped from a plastic cup of water, and
my voice was a frail, ragged whisper. I did my best to answer the
host's questions, as well as those of the guests who called in,
though I can't recall a word I said. All I remember was pressing the
button on the control board, aptly labeled COUGH, to mute the
sounds of my phlegmatic hacking as my lungs gasped for air. I
must have pressed that button fifty times.

By the end of the interview, I was slouched in my chair, wrecked
from the exertion of having to talk and sit upright. The host had
one final question. "We just have a few seconds left," he said. "Are
you facing mortality at this point?"

I was thrown. My mortality was something I'd logged a lot of
time thinking about, of course, but this was the first time anyone
had asked me this question outright. Hearing it posed out loud, on
national radio, made the threat of death feel more vivid and imminent than it had ever been. It made me realize that the host, the
listeners, the people who read my column—they were all probably
wondering the same thing: Would I live or would I die? My survival had inadvertently become narrative suspense; strangers followed my story with a morbid curiosity about what the next weeks
would bring. The thought unsettled me. I steeled myself, determined to end the interview on a strong note, but when I spoke, my
voice sounded crepe-thin. "I feel very hopeful for the future," I
whispered unconvincingly.

Whatever was brewing in my lungs that day quickly overtook
my immune system. That weekend, on Mother's Day, instead of
eating brunch and watching a movie with my mom in the lounge
of the Hope Lodge as we had planned, I was curled up on a
stretcher in the emergency room, with her by my side. My blood

pressure was bottoming out, and my heart rate was dangerously high. Despite my protests, the doctors readmitted me to the hospital. "I jinxed myself," I told my mother, recalling my final words from the radio interview. "I should have said I feel *cautiously* hopeful for the future."

We are born needing care and we die needing care, but it was hard for me to accept how helpless I'd become. Back at the Hope Lodge, after a fog of touch-and-go days in the hospital, I was as weak as ever, reduced to a toddler-like dependency on Will and my mother. In the weeks that followed, I grew weaker, and by Day 70, I needed their help with even the most basic tasks like showering and making a sandwich. Too frail and nauseated to walk, I used a wheelchair to get around. In the middle of the night I would wake up and feel my heart's unsteady beat against my chest, lagging and quickening in a way that unsettled me and made me hyperaware of my own vulnerability.

Then, around Day 80, a dusky rash appeared on my forehead, and everyone went into a panic. This was the first symptom of GVHD, the potentially deadly complication of transplant I had been warned about. My doctors ramped up my dosage of the steroids and antirejection drugs and monitored me closely, hoping for the best.

My independence wasn't the only thing I could feel slipping away. Ever since moving into the Hope Lodge, Will had started coming home from work later and later each night. He'd call at the last minute to ask if someone could take the evening shift, and if I said that it might be difficult on such short notice, he'd ask why we didn't have more support. I knew the Hope Lodge wasn't the most fun place to hang out and that my body's demands were taxing. I had no energy to give him, and yet I needed him more than ever. When we were together, I soaked up his love like a sponge, desperate to feel close again. When I brought up his growing distance, Will insisted it was all in my head. Still, I worried.

One night, as I waited for Will to return from work, I received a text from him: *I'm getting drinks at a bar on Saint Marks with some friends. Want to come?* I stared at my phone, wondering how to respond. He may have genuinely wanted me there, but we both knew I was many weeks, probably months, away from being well enough to go anywhere in public. Let alone a bar on Saint Marks, one of the grimiest, most crowded places in all of lower Manhattan. As I attempted to compose a reply, tears clotted my eyes. I dug my nails into my palms, ordering myself not to cry. *Sorry, I can't. But I think you know that,* I texted back. My mother was putting on her coat and getting ready to head out for the night. It was a rare evening when she had dinner plans with a friend, and although I knew she would have been more than happy to stay with me, I didn't ask.

Alone in my twin bed, I waited for Will. Night swooped down, submerging the room in darkness, and the city lights shone brightly outside the window. As the hours passed, a cold, visceral dread welled in my gut. I needed to eat something before taking the last of my medications, but I was too weak to walk to the communal kitchen down the hall, so I washed the handful of pills down with water. An amateur's mistake. By the time Will came home, it was past midnight. I was doubled over a wastebasket, the sheets around me soiled in vomit, my pajamas drenched in sweat. He froze at the foot of my bed, guilt washing over his face. As he scooped me into his arms and carried me to the shower, I felt two competing emotions duking it out in my heart: *I hate you, I need you.*

It was the morning of Day 100. I sat in one of the blue plastic booths in the communal kitchen as Will prepared breakfast. To appease him, I pushed a lump of congealing oatmeal around with a spoon, pretending to eat, but my thoughts were elsewhere. In a few minutes we would leave for the hospital to receive the results of the various tests and biopsies I'd undergone in the last week. In my mind there were two potential outcomes: The results would show either that the transplant had worked and I would eventually be okay, or that the transplant had failed and the leukemia would return, this time with the promise of imminent death. It never occurred to me that there might be a third possibility.

As Will did the dishes, I scrolled anxiously through unread emails from readers, searching for a distraction. One, in particular, caught my eye. The subject line read: *the difficulty of transitioning back*. Attached to the email was a photograph of a young man sitting shirtless in a hospital room. He had broad, muscular shoulders, and his rosy cheeks emanated a seemingly radioactive glow. His head, like mine, was smooth and bald, but I was struck by how confident he seemed. I handed my phone to Will to show him the photograph. Will whistled. "Damn. He looks better than I do. If I didn't know any better, I'd worry that you'd found yourself a cancer boyfriend to replace me."

The young man's name was Ned. His email opened with a story. Back in 2010, Ned had been midway through his senior year of college, blissfully unaware of what awaited him on the other side of graduation. He was busy writing his honors thesis and had just started dating a beautiful girl. He'd submitted a Fulbright application to Italy, where he hoped to live after graduation. Then, while home in Boston during winter break, he got a CT scan that showed that his spleen was enlarged. After some more tests, the doctors confirmed that he had leukemia. It wasn't the first time Ned had gotten sick. Three years earlier, he had been diagnosed with testicular cancer, but he mentioned this as an afterthought. *"Cancer-lite," all I needed was a surgery,* was how he put it.

It was a story I knew well. It was my story. It was the story of the countless other young cancer patients whom I'd heard from since the column's launch, stories that had brought me comfort, showing me just how many of us there were out there, an invisible community, hidden from sight in hospital rooms and chained to IV poles.

But then Ned's story veered in an unexpected direction. *What inspired me to write you is something that I know you'll be covering soon enough—transitioning back to the real world, "normality,"* he wrote. *I've been having a hard time getting back on the horse.* When I read that, I realized that this wasn't a letter about cancer in youth. It was about what happened once the cancer was gone. The notion of a life after cancer wasn't something I could entertain, at least not yet. I was still stuck in the Hope Lodge; still using a wheelchair to get around; still far too sick to contemplate anything other than my impending bone marrow biopsy results— let alone the notion of a life after cancer.

A few minutes later, Will and I went down to the lobby of the Hope Lodge. My mother was waiting there for us, and together we went out, hailed a taxi, then climbed in. I had brought with me a couple of plastic bags in case I got sick during the ride over, but this time it was nerves, not nausea, that made my stomach churn. When we reached the hospital, we rode the elevator up to the out-patient bone marrow transplant unit in silence, too anxious to talk.

The receptionist called my name and we were ushered to a room in the back of the clinic. I held my breath as my medical team entered, a nurse practitioner followed by my transplant doctor, who was stout and spectacled and sported a perpetually stern expression that masked a gentle disposition. "The good news is that your latest biopsy shows no cancerous cells in your bone marrow," he said. "The transplant appears to be working—for now— but it'll be many more months and many more diagnostic days like this one, before we can know for sure."

"The bad news?" I asked. Of course, I hoped that there wouldn't be any, but by this point I knew enough about the way doctors framed these types of conversations to suspect that wasn't the case.

"Well, the bad news is that you are at a high risk of relapse. Because of the chromosomal abnormalities in your marrow and the fact that we weren't able to fully get rid of the leukemia before the transplant, your disease has a strong likelihood of coming back. I'd like for you to begin an experimental maintenance chemo regimen right away, as soon as you are strong enough."

Sitting on the exam table, I hugged my knees to my chest. I was engulfed by despair. It was the kind of despair that felt like drowning and made voices sound small and distant, as if underwater. My mind flashed to parts of Ned's letter from earlier that morning. *What could possibly be so hard about transitioning back to normality?* I thought bitterly now. *All I want is normality. I'll be lucky to ever leave these hospital rooms.* My cancer was a junkyard dog. It may have been fenced in for now, but it was mean and growling, threatening to dig under the barbed wire and escape. I would have to fight like hell to keep it behind the fence. I'd have to endure more experimental treatments and after that countless tests, over months and years, tracking progress to a cure. There would always be another scan down the road. The biopsy next time.

"How long will I have to do the maintenance chemo?" I asked my transplant doctor, bracing for the response. "A long time," he said softly. "Another year, possibly more." I looked at Will. His face had taken on the sunken, despondent quality of a man who was trapped. I couldn't blame him. And yet, looking back, I see now that I did.

17

CHRONOLOGY OF FREEDOM

HOME IS AN elusive concept for people like me. By the time I was twelve, I'd attended six schools on three different continents. From seventh grade onward, we'd stayed put in Saratoga, for the most part, but I never grew to feel like I was *from* there, or anywhere else for that matter. I got antsy when I stayed in the same place for longer than a year or two, afraid of getting stuck, like a barnacle to the hull of a ship. This is the curse of the mixed child who grows up betwixt cultures and countries, creeds and customs: too white, too brown, too exotically named, too ambiguously other to ever fully belong anywhere.

Life since diagnosis had been no less nomadic. In the last year, Will and I had spent a combined total of six months living out of hospital rooms. We'd lived in my childhood bedroom in Saratoga. We'd lived in the guest bedrooms of friends. And most recently, we'd been living at the Hope Lodge, where the rules mandated we could stay for a maximum of three months. But by the end of summer, I was cured of my transient tendencies. More than anything, I yearned for a home.

In late August of 2012, Will and I relocated to the apartment my mother owned on the corner of Fourth Street and Avenue A in the East Village—the same apartment where, two decades earlier, she had lived when she first immigrated to New York. As long as Will and I could come up with enough to cover the maintenance, utilities, and taxes, the apartment was ours for however long we wanted to stay.

So much had changed since I'd last visited the building, but so very little. When I arrived I heard someone call out, *"Le bébé!"* and saw Jorge, who worked as the doorman in the evenings. He was now an old man, gray and slightly hunched, but he still remembered the day my parents brought me home from the hospital as a newborn. All the doors in the building were still painted the same shade of seafoam green, the hallways were adorned with faux gold moldings and art deco light fixtures. The elevator broke down on the regular and the faucets occasionally spouted rust-brown water. The matchbox-sized apartment was located on the ground floor, with windows that looked onto the dumpsters in the courtyard. Will's parents bought us a dish rack and glasses, mine loaned us bedding and a beautiful old Tunisian rug, and a friend gave us a bed frame. We had also scoured thrift stores for an old steamer trunk, like the one we'd used as our dining table in Paris. A home, no matter how small, dimly lit, or haphazardly furnished, meant a new kind of freedom, and we felt wildly lucky.

On our first night in the apartment, Will set two plates on the trunk and lit some candles. The last real, full meal I remembered being able to eat was an Easter dinner in the transplant unit, and until recently my food had come via tubes or through the small bites of overcooked fare I'd managed to stomach at the Hope Lodge. My weight was at an all-time low and I had zero appetite, but I was determined to enjoy our first dinner in our new home.

Freedom meant being able to eat half a bowl of homemade spaghetti—and then fighting all night to keep it down.

Freedom also meant being patient with Will in the weeks that followed, as he struggled to fill the shoes of the hospital staff and my mother, who had returned to Saratoga. He took on the bulk of the household chores, cooking and cleaning, and accompanied me to the emergency room when, every few weeks, I came down with another fever or faced some new complication. I was so weak that even walking to the pharmacy one block away was a challenge, so I spent most days alone in bed, sleeping, trying to write, and numbing out on television. I counted down the hours until noon, when Will would bike home during his lunch break to check up on me and fix me something to eat before returning to work. And then I counted down the hours until seven, when he came home. Since I still wasn't allowed to go out to crowded places, eat restaurant food, or take public transportation, in the evenings we stayed in. The distance I'd felt from him in the Hope Lodge had lessened. Both of us were giddy about the prospect of starting afresh in a place of our own. Freedom meant being able to share a bed together for the first time since the transplant, and reckoning with a new body that seemed to have forgotten how to speak the language of physical intimacy.

It was a Monday morning, just past nine o'clock. I was standing outside the apartment building, and someone was trying to hail a taxi on each corner. I sat down on the curb and figured I'd wait a few minutes for the morning commute rush to calm. I had started chemo again, and no matter what I did—skip the shower, set multiple alarms, go to sleep early the night before—I always seemed to arrive at the hospital exactly thirty minutes late. I wasn't in a huge hurry—my thirty-minute lateness buffer had become so consistent, I was almost proud of it. I was on time, but it was my time.

Maybe I was also secretly hoping that if I showed up late enough, I'd be told I could take the day off. I strained against having to do the maintenance chemo at all. Now that I had no blast counts—no cancer, only the threat of its return—it was harder for me to rally my resolve and submit to the torturous process, even if my logical mind understood the reasons why. My new treatment regimen entailed an intravenous infusion of azacitidine, a drug I'd taken during the clinical trial. I would receive it for five consecutive days each month. Then I would have three weeks off. On paper, it sounded like no big deal. But my experience had taught me that the time off would be no vacation—I'd slog through those three weeks, leadened by the toxic chemicals, then, just as I'd start to feel better, it would be time for another five days. This was my life for the foreseeable future.

A taxi slowed, and I halfheartedly waved it down. The driver was an older man with salt-and-pepper twists and a heavy Jamaican accent. As we sped up the FDR Drive, the highway that runs along the eastern edge of Manhattan, I caught a glimpse of a young woman cycling on the bike path along the East River. She looked about my age, tan, athletic, her blond ponytail dancing in the wind. Someday, maybe I'd ride a bike to the hospital, I thought. Once I was well enough.

"Hel-lo? Anyone home?" said the taxi driver. We'd arrived at the hospital, and I had been lost in my thoughts. "Everything okay?" I had this running joke in my head that one day, when someone asked me how I was doing, I'd unload a monologue about my latest cytogenetic report or biopsy results, just to see how they'd react. But the driver was just trying to be nice. I knew he didn't actually want me to explain how a bone marrow transplant can leave a person disoriented and scatterbrained. Or that I'd become quasi-narcoleptic in public. So instead I kept my mouth shut, paid the fare, and exited the cab with a quick "thanks."

The familiar scent of antiseptic stung my nostrils as I stepped into the main lobby of Sloan Kettering. With its twenty floors, sparkling steel elevators, and walls lined with artwork, it resembled a giant cruise ship packed with cancer patients and the people who cared for them. It even had the weird, scaled-down amenities of a cruise: a Starbucks cart, a dining hall, the occasional chamber music concert, and a recreation floor, with arts and crafts activities and a library where patients could check out battered copies of Harlequin Romance novels. The building was spotless and equipped with state-of-the-art equipment, but there was a weariness, bordering on shabbiness, throughout. The waiting rooms were decorated with seventies-style furniture and the marbled linoleum floors were worn where doctors and caregivers had paced over the years. The urgent care unit was always at capacity and patients in wheelchairs and stretchers overflowed into the hallway.

The first time I visited Sloan Kettering was a few days after my diagnosis, when I'd come seeking a second opinion. With my waist-length hair and nose ring, I didn't look like the other patients. In the waiting room, a middle-aged man with a sleeveless shirt and a bandana covering his hairless head had leaned in toward my father, who has been bald since the nineties, and, assuming he was the one undergoing chemo, raised his fist in the air. "Live strong, brother," he said. I remember feeling vindicated, as though the mix-up was proof that I didn't belong here—that I was somehow different from these patients in their various stages of decay. Now I found the patients and the sterile scent of Sloan Kettering soothing. With my quarter inch of duckling blond hair, patchily growing in and soft as down, I fit in and felt at ease here. I understood the protocols, spoke fluent medicalese, and could navigate the complex web of hallways with my eyes closed. It was the outside world that had grown foreign, even a little frightening.

I pumped the hand sanitizer dispenser three times—my good luck ritual—and rubbed my palms together, then pulled on a pair of blue latex gloves and a fresh face mask, and marched to the B elevators. I shivered when the doors opened onto the fourth floor. The outpatient bone marrow transplant clinic was kept airless and cold, like a meat locker. I swiped a heated blanket from the nurses' station—an oven-like contraption there kept them toasty warm—and took a seat.

The hours spent sitting around in waiting rooms seemed endless, best passed in a state of stillness, or people watching. Over time, I'd become an expert in recognizing the different phases of Patienthood: The newly diagnosed were often accompanied by an entourage of friends and relatives carrying flowers and gifts; some semi-balding father or son with an already low-stakes hair situation would shave his head in solidarity, believing he deserved a badge of honor for this sacrifice. After a few weeks, the entourage would thin. A calendar designating "Chemo Buddy Duty" would be drafted so that friends and family could take turns accompanying the patient. Within six months, the patient would be sitting next to a single caregiver, whose heavy responsibilities left them grumbling about the parking situation or the "hellish wait times." If the patient had the misfortune of being sick for longer than a year or two, it would eventually be determined that they could handle coming to the hospital alone.

Today, for the first time since my diagnosis, I had joined the ranks of the latter—however, I wasn't the only one. I noticed a young man who'd just entered and was donning the requisite mask and gloves. He looked to be in his late twenties, tall and lanky with a wool hat covering his head. He seemed nervous as he scanned the crowded waiting room for a place to sit. The only empty chair happened to be directly to my right and we nodded at each other as he approached.

"Suleika, right?" he said, extending a gloved hand. "I'm a big fan of your column." He introduced himself as Bret, and as we waited, he told me about what he described as a losing battle with lymphoma, and how he and his wife were considering uprooting their lives in Chicago to move here, to New York City, so that he could undergo a bone marrow transplant. I listened, then shared with him the relevant parts of my experience. I told him that he'd be well taken care of if he decided to have his transplant here, and I also offered to connect him to the Hope Lodge, where he and his wife could live free of charge. By the time Bret's name was called, his hands were steady, and I felt grounded by our conversation— our connection. We exchanged phone numbers, and I promised to look him up if I was ever in Chicago. But once he disappeared behind the curtain, I was on my own again.

When I was finally called into the chemo suite, I saw Abbie, one of my favorite nurses. "Your eyes are red," she said, with a hint of concern. "I'm just tired," I began to say—and that was partially true. I hadn't been sleeping so well lately. The high dose of steroids I took to fight the GVHD gave me insomnia, and I'd stay up late watching movies in bed. But before I could say anything else, I found myself full-on weeping. The outburst surprised me. At home, I had turned into a walking tear fountain, but I rarely did so in front of others.

My spirit had been troubled waters lately—churning, uneasy— ever since I'd found out I would need to do more chemo. With Will busy at work and my parents back home in Saratoga, freedom was learning to care for myself. It was an enormous pillbox labeled with the days of the week, and the responsibility to take the dozens of medications on time. Freedom was going solo to chemo. It was the realization that I was in this alone. In a sense, I always had been.

18

THE MUTT

AS A KID, while my brother and our friends were busy climbing trees and chasing soccer balls, I scoured the sidewalks and bushes for abandoned animals. I never passed a discarded cardboard box or a dumpster without peeking inside, checking for litters of kittens that had been tossed away with the trash. When adults asked me what I wanted to be when I grew up, I replied with all the earnestness in the world: the Mother Teresa of strays.

All those years, I begged my parents for a puppy, but they said no every time—we moved around too much, and they didn't want the extra responsibility. Every day after school in the fourth and fifth grades, I rode my bike to the local animal hospital, where I helped clean kennels, observed surgeries, and restocked the supply closets. I spent my allowance on old veterinary science textbooks as well as kibble, kitten formula, and toys to donate to animal rescue organizations. I memorized all 274 dog breeds recognized by the American Kennel Club and forced my parents to quiz me on their behavioral traits, health needs, and life expectancies. When I was ten, I asked my brother for an incubator for Christmas. By spring, to my parents' dismay, I was carting around a dozen baby chicks in my old doll stroller. After that came the hamster-breeding business followed by a pet-sitting side hustle. In middle school I made weekend pilgrimages to the animal shelter, where I spent my days communing with mangy old dogs. I especially liked the mutts—the scruffier, more mischievous and feral, more utterly untrainable the better. On some level, I think I related to them—they were outsiders, searching for a home.

I clung to this calling for a while longer, fostering a newborn kitten that I named Mohamed for a brief time in college. But I was busy with classes and soon had to hand him over to a more reliable owner. As time passed, there was summer travel, orchestra rehearsals, boyfriends, and parties. After graduation, there was no room in my adult life for a pet. I could barely take care of myself.

A therapy dog had come to visit me in the early days of my diagnosis back at Mount Sinai, a small energetic spaniel that had jumped around on my hospital bed, playfully tugging at the blanket on my lap. For the first time since falling ill, I didn't feel like I was being treated as if I were made of porcelain. The visit with the therapy dog sparked a renewed wave of pleading for a pet, just as I'd done as a kid, and ever since moving into the apartment with Will, I'd become even more fixated on the idea. I spent hours on my computer scrolling through animal adoption websites. But I knew the medical reality: My weakened immune system made getting a dog impossible. My transplant doctor didn't think twice about rejecting the prospect. Still I made a point of asking every few weeks.

One October morning, while at Sloan Kettering for a checkup, I learned that my transplant doctor had taken a short-term medical leave. In his absence, I was being reassigned to a different doctor, named—quite auspiciously—Dr. Barker. With her, I decided to try my luck.

"What do you think about me getting a dog?" I asked within minutes of our first appointment.

She mulled it over for a moment. "Sure," Dr. Barker replied. "I don't see why not." She pointed out that my immune system was stronger—not as strong as it could be, but strong enough—and caring for a pet might even be therapeutic, she said.

I didn't waste much time. Later that afternoon, I convinced Will to take me to a rescue animal organization in SoHo after work—"just to look." I went straight for the runt. He was an ugly terrier mash-up—a "schnoodle," part schnauzer, part poodle—with sparse white fur that barely concealed his mottled purplish flesh and floppy ears. I couldn't resist and asked to hold him. He was small enough that he fit into the palm of my hand. Growling, with a scruffy goatee and a mischievous glint in his eyes, he looked grumpy and slightly unhinged, but full of character. It was love at first sight. "That's my dog," I said.

Will was apprehensive, worried about the exposure to germs and the added burden of caring for a pet when we were already up against more than we could handle. I begged, promising to take precautions to protect my health and coming up with an inexhaustible flow of solutions: The dog would wear disposable booties on walks to keep his paws as unsoiled as possible. I vowed to wear gloves when feeding and cleaning up after him, swore that he would never sleep in the bed, and made a list of four friends who could help take care of him when I lacked the energy.

"You are relentless," Will said with a hint of a smile.

When I told the woman at the desk that we were interested in adopting the runt, she said that there was a wait list of a dozen people ahead of us who'd already put down applications for the same puppy. She would need to review all of the applications and to call everyone's references before a decision could be made. I hesitated for a moment, then implored, "Any idea when we might expect to hear back? I was hoping to get the puppy before my next round of chemo. You know what they say . . . dogs are the best medicine." It was the first and only time I would ever play the cancer card, but I desperately wanted the runt. Clearly moved by the intensity of my performance, the woman practically thrust the adoption papers at us. In the taxi ride back to our apartment, the runt became "Oscar."

That first night with Oscar was the happiest I could remember since my diagnosis. Within an hour, he had peed twice and taken a shit of shocking proportions on the old Tunisian rug in our living room, but I was too smitten to care. Will quickly got into the spirit of things and together we gave him a bath, fawning over him like ecstatic new parents. When Oscar finally crashed on my chest, I rubbed his belly and watched him sleep, his tiny black paws twitching as he chased rabbits through dreams. The warmth of his body and the steady beat of his heart against my chest relaxed me, and I fell asleep on the couch, with Oscar curled under my arm.

Reality set in the next day when Will went off to work and I found myself alone with Oscar for the first time. I was not prepared for the task of sprinting outside half a dozen times a day, carrying an incontinent puppy, an arc of urine splattering the hallway floors before I could reach the doors. The chemo and transplant had left me devoid of energy, and I still needed so much rest. But Oscar didn't give a damn if I was too nauseated or in pain to play fetch. Caring for him quickly became the most dreaded part of my day. Every morning, after Will left for work, Oscar would begin the process of baptizing my toes with his tongue until I woke up. Then off for a walk. After a few blocks, he was warmed up and ready for a run, whereas I was exhausted and ready to crawl back into bed. I wondered if I'd made a huge mistake.

But slowly, in time, the two of us started to get our acts together. Living with Oscar left me no choice but to develop a structure to my days that revolved around his needs rather than my own. Oscar stopped using the living room rug as his personal pee pad, and I stopped sleeping in until noon. Oscar finished getting his booster shots, and I got all of my childhood vaccinations for the second time. (A patient's childhood immunizations are lost during a bone marrow transplant.) Trying to keep up with Oscar also turned out to be good rehab. My muscles had atrophied from spending so much time on bed rest, but within a few weeks of being forced to take multiple walks a day, we were bounding up and down stairs, taking them two by two.

For the first time in a long time, it wasn't cancer that dominated my days. "Okay, buddy," I said, clapping my hands as I called Oscar for his walk. "Lead the way." He leaped ahead, tugging at the leash as he guided me out of the apartment building and toward the dog run in Tompkins Square Park, where we'd made lots of new friends. There was Mochi, the terrier mix who liked to wrestle in the sand with Oscar; Thelma and Louise, the shy brother and sister beagle duo who preferred to watch the other dogs play from a distance; and Max, the giant coonhound, whose favorite activity was attacking the fur trim on women's coats. Rather than stare at the poor girl in the face mask, passersby stopped to pet Oscar and to tell me how cute he was. The other tenants in my building now said hello to my dog before greeting me. And instead of discussing my symptoms and treatment plan for the week, Will and I were busy with potty training and obedience classes. It was nice not to be the center of attention for a change.

I was still in a tenuous type of remission reserved for "high risk" leukemia patients in their first year out of transplant. I still took twenty-three pills a day and spent most hours—both sleeping and awake—in bed. I still had weekly checkups at the hospital, and I still felt anxious at each appointment, as I waited to hear that my blood counts were all right. And once a month, I still did a five-day course of chemo. Oscar couldn't change what was going on in my marrow, but he was working a different kind of magic. Since adopting him, I'd felt a burst of energy, a glimmer of being normal again.

19

DREAMING IN WATERCOLOR

BEING IN A hospital can feel a lot like living in a big city. Activity swirls around you as patients walk the hallways, residents make their morning rounds, nurses chat in clusters by the coffee machine. Still, you can feel profoundly isolated, alienated.

Without a caregiver to accompany me to appointments anymore, the hours of tedium were relieved only by the messages from readers that continued to flood my in-box. Since the launch of "Life, Interrupted," it had been syndicated in magazines and newspapers and was gaining a sizable following. I didn't have the stamina to write a new column each week, but I did keep writing, slowly, every day, even if it was only a paragraph. Other than the occasional waiting room chitchat or sidewalk hellos, I never thought to take encounters with readers any further. But I was starved for conversation with someone I could relate to, for an antidote to the loneliness. As I sat in the waiting room, preparing to begin my third cycle of the maintenance chemo, I read a Facebook message from a young woman by the name of Melissa Carroll, who was also undergoing treatment at Sloan Kettering. I responded, asking if she wanted to get together, and she replied a few minutes later, saying she was also at the hospital that day and asked if I wanted to hang out.

After I finished my chemo in the bone marrow transplant clinic, I took the elevator upstairs to eat lunch with Melissa during her infusion. At thirty, Melissa was one of the oldest patients in the pediatric cancer ward. She had Ewing sarcoma, a vicious type of bone cancer that typically affects toddlers and teens, which was how she had ended up on the ninth floor.

The pediatric ward was a world unto itself. The walls were decorated with painted murals and cheery paper cutouts of animals. The fluorescent lights, harsh and unflattering elsewhere in the hospital, were warmer here, casting a cozy glow. It was the week before Halloween, and all of the doctors and nurses had dressed up in costume. Even the face masks were hooked up—they came in every color of the rainbow and some had smiley faces and mustaches painted on them. Opposite the reception desk was an enormous rectangular playpen filled with toys, games, dollhouses, and stuffed animals. A girl, no older than five, with translucent skin and a thin scar that snaked down the center of her skull, pushed a doll in and out of a wooden box. When I looked more closely, I saw that the box was a toy CT scan machine. Next to the girl, a nurse sat cross-legged, quietly explaining to her how it worked, like a warped version of preschool.

My quest in the last few months had been to become an adult, as if adulthood were a test I could study for, fill in the right answers, and ace. I was twenty-four years old. I had a puppy to raise, bills to pay, and columns to churn out. I had a boyfriend whom I was going to marry once I was done with treatment, and I went to my chemo appointments all by myself. But standing there among the brightly painted walls and jars of lollipops, I wished badly that I could be in pediatrics, where I was closer in age to many of the patients, rather than downstairs in the bone marrow transplant clinic with the early bird dinner crowd.

I walked around the playpen to the far side of the ward, where Melissa sat in one of the La-Z-Boy-style recliners, facing a row of windows. Her long dark wig, which she curled into soft waves, was a startling contrast to her parchment-pale skin and rose-painted lips. But it was her eyes—enormous, with irises like green sea glass, fringed by long black lashes—that made her face impossible to forget. An IV bag hung above her, drip-dropping poison into her tattooed arms. She clapped her hands together and smiled when she spotted me. "Suleika!" she said with a slight lisp. We didn't hug, abiding by the strict no-contact rule between immuno-compromised patients. "It's cool here, right?" she said. "There's a lot of light."

I settled into the recliner next to her, and when lunchtime came, we ordered the star-shaped peanut butter and jelly sandwiches—Melissa said they were her favorite item on the kids' menu. We looked out the windows as we ate, and I asked her dozens of questions, wanting to know everything about my mysterious new hospital buddy. Melissa told me about how she was born in Ireland, where her dad, a musician, was from, but had grown up in a small town in New Hampshire. She told me about learning to play the drums in her early teenage years and about the short-lived all-girl indie rock band she started called Mystic Spiral. After graduating from art school, Melissa had moved to Brooklyn, where she'd spent five years working as an assistant to Francesco Clemente, a famous contemporary painter.

"Twenty ten was a good year for me," Melissa said, her eyes filled with longing. She had a boyfriend and a buzzing social life, and her paintings were beginning to show in galleries. Then, one night, she met up with a friend for drinks in Williamsburg, and in the dark of the bar her friend had accidentally squashed her foot with the steel leg of a stool. At first, Melissa thought she had suffered a sprain, but weeks later the pain was still there, and a hard knobby bump had appeared on the top of her foot. Melissa, who at the time didn't have insurance, had finally found a sliding-scale clinic, and an X-ray showed a crushed third metatarsal bone. It also showed that the lump wasn't just swelling but an abnormal mass. A biopsy revealed the mass was malignant, and that the cancer had already spread to her pelvic lymph nodes and knee. "You don't get cancer from a barstool, obviously," Melissa said. "If my friend hadn't squashed my foot in that exact location, I probably wouldn't have discovered the cancer. Pretty wild, right?"

After the diagnosis, Melissa had no choice but to move back to New Hampshire to live with her parents. She began an intensive regimen of chemo and when her hair started to fall out, she locked herself in the bathroom and shaved her head with clippers. Afterward, her mom drove her to a salon in Boston to be fitted for a wig that looked identical to her inky black locks streaked with chestnut highlights. That same night, she put it on, boarded a train back to New York, and went to a party in Bushwick. "I showed my friends the wig and then jumped right into the backyard swimming pool," she told me with an irreverent smirk. That was Melissa: effervescent and fun-loving, quick to laugh and always smiling, even in the grimmest of circumstances. In her presence, things brightened and opened up.

This was Melissa's second time in treatment. She had undergone seventeen cycles of chemo and multiple surgeries the first time, and at the end of that, her scans came back clear. But only a year and a half after her diagnosis, her cancer was back, and she'd decided to transfer her care to Sloan Kettering, where more treatment options were available. When she got the news of the relapse, she was devastated and she sat down on her parents' porch and opened her sketchbook. She had previously worked with oil paints on large canvases but the fumes now made her sick, so she began to experiment with watercolors and made her first in a series of haunting paintings, entitled *Self-Portrait with Mask*. "I like the uncertainty and the happy accidents that you get with watercolors. I like how you don't have total control, like life," she told me. "Maybe you could come over sometime and I could paint your portrait?"

I nodded eagerly. Melissa was someone I would have hung out with before my diagnosis, and I was thrilled to have made a new friend who was also trying to find ways to creatively engage with illness. We were both forging unlikely careers: Melissa painted self-portraits from bed; I wrote self-portraits from bed. Watercolors and words were the drugs we preferred for our pain. We were learning that sometimes the only way to endure suffering is to transform it into art.

Melissa and I soon became inseparable. We kept each other company during chemo. We spent afternoons scouring thrift stores for matching leather jackets and new threads that fit our skeletal frames. In the evenings, we hung out at her apartment in Brooklyn, which overlooked McGolrick Park and was decorated with a baffling collection of knickknacks: a taxidermied two-headed duckling sent to her by one of her many suitors, a beautiful glass bong, a wooden crate filled with dozens of pill bottles and paintbrushes, and a giant corkboard on one wall, where she'd tacked hospital bracelets, photographs of friends, old plane tickets, and past career accolades. To ward off the nausea she smoked pot constantly and when she got the munchies fixed us bowls of ice cream. She let me borrow one of her wigs and gave me makeup tutorials, teaching me how to pencil in my eyebrows and paste thick rows of fake eyelashes where mine had fallen out. Melissa loved to dance, and when we had the energy, we would blast *Thriller* on the speakers and twirl around the living room, whipping our wigs around to the beat until we collapsed on the couch.

One topic that came up a lot during our endless chats was love. Finding love during a prolonged illness—let alone holding on to that love—was daunting. Sometimes, it could seem straight-up impossible. I was one of the rare young adult patients whose significant other had stuck around during treatment. "Hold on to him," Melissa would often say. "You don't know how lucky you are." A few months after her diagnosis, her longtime boyfriend had dumped her, moved to the West Coast, and promptly fallen into a new relationship with a much younger woman. "A world-class asshole," Melissa said.

But the topic we liked to talk about more than any other was all the places we would travel once we were better. We planned itineraries to faraway lands. Melissa dreamed of palm trees and spice markets, rickshaws and elephants. I imagined myself reporting from some distant locale, or speeding down the California coast in a beat-up convertible. People often described cancer as a journey. But we didn't want to go on some bullshit "cancer journey"—we wanted to go on a *real* journey, one that would rocket us from the cancer ward's sounds, smells, and sad plastic plants, and plunge us into the reckless lives we wished we were living.

Two skinny girls, all elbows and knees, protruding cheekbones, and buzzed heads full of desperate dreams for the future—any future, as long as we could be there.

Later that winter, a few months after we met, Melissa found out that her cancer had spread to her lungs. She responded by buying a plane ticket to India. "Less bucket list, more fuck-it list," she explained, sitting at her kitchen table as she sucked on a joint. While surfing the Internet, she had discovered A Fresh Chapter, a nonprofit that offers trips abroad and volunteer opportunities for cancer survivors with the intent of helping them find new meaning and direction after treatment. "India has always been my dream— the colors, the culture, make me want to paint," Melissa said.

"Cancer has taken so much from me and I need this. I just want to feel inspired again."

My eyes widened with concern as I thought about her going to a country where even healthy travelers are known to get sick. "But what if you come down with a neutropenic fever?" I asked. "What if you need to be hospitalized while you're there?"

"What's the worst that can happen?" she replied. "Suleika, for the first time, I feel like I'm going to die. I am going to die from this fucking disease."

We sat very still, a heavy silence thickening the air around us.

Too sick to travel anywhere outside of a fifty-mile radius of the hospital, let alone join her in India, I cheered Melissa on from my bed when she left that March, living vicariously through the photographs and the updates she sent me by text every couple of days. For two glorious weeks, Melissa wasn't a cancer patient—she got to be Melissa the Artist who taught drawing and painting classes through a volunteer program at an elementary school in Delhi. She stopped at the Lotus Temple and said a heartfelt prayer. In one of the many outdoor markets, she came across gorgeous hand-painted marionettes and bought so many she needed a second suitcase to bring them home. The highlight of her trip was a visit to the Taj Mahal, which was more beautiful than anything she had ever seen. Traveling to India, she had eluded for a brief moment the specter of her own mortality. One day I picked up my phone and saw a message from her that said, *I've never felt more alive.*

Meanwhile, in New York, the city had been knocked flat by a blizzard. Great swaths of snow fell from the sky, padding the sidewalks and trees and buildings in a heavy blanket of white, soon tracked with shoe prints but still lovely. I closed the drapes, but the streetlamps refracted off the snow, basking the apartment in a watery blue light. Will had inherited an old television from a friend, and he'd set it up on a card table so that we could watch movies in bed. It was a Sunday night and we lounged side by side, me with a heating pad on my stomach, him with a can of beer that he drained in long gulps.

When Will stood up to grab another beer, I resisted the urge to tell him to slow down, not wanting to further irk him or become the kind of nagging girlfriend who might appear in a sitcom. Something was weighing on him, but I was afraid to ask what it was because I was pretty sure the answer had to do with me. Lately, when he returned from work, he seemed restless and frustrated. He would sigh if I asked him to walk the dog or to run an errand, and he made little reproachful comments about how he wished he had more time to himself or to hang out with friends. I hated how much I needed from him, and it was humiliating to ask someone for help when you had the sense they didn't really want to give it. After I fell asleep, I would sometimes hear the furtive closing of a door, and I would get up to discover that he had left for a walk or to go watch a game at the sports bar next door. I'd lie awake, waiting for him to return, waiting for the sun to rise, waiting out the tension that had slowly infiltrated our relationship like mold.

"We need more help," Will would say again and again. Tasked with the role of boyfriend, caregiver, and normal twentysomething trying to figure out who he was and what he wanted to do with his life, Will was overwhelmed, buckling under the weight of his many responsibilities. He never said it outright, but it was clear that he was getting fed up with the limitations and demands my health placed upon us.

"So, a couple of people from work are going to a music festival in Texas tomorrow," Will told me when he returned from the kitchen with his beer. "I was thinking of maybe buying a last-minute plane ticket and joining them for a couple of days." His tone was casual, but his face was tensely composed.

"I have chemo this week and surgery on Friday." I was getting a port to replace the catheter I had ripped from my chest. "I need you here." The desperation in my tone made me cringe.

"I know, I know, and I'm sorry," Will said, "but I really need a break. And maybe, while I'm there, I can do some writing of my own."

I wanted to be the graceful leukemic starlet who told him, *Take as many breaks as you want, you deserve it, have a wonderful trip, my love,* but there is a spiritual exhaustion that comes with maintaining this kind of charade after a while. As a patient, there was pressure to perform, to be someone who suffers well, to act with heroism, and to put on a stoic façade all the time. But that night, I didn't have it in me to listen to how hard my illness was on Will—how badly he needed a break when I didn't have the option of taking a break from this body, from this disease, from this life of ours.

"Why do you take breaks in the moments when I need you most?" I asked, although the question was mostly rhetorical.

"There's always something going wrong with you," Will said. "When is it ever a good time?"

My vision shuddered in and out of focus, like the beginning of a violent migraine. Without realizing what I was doing, I reached for a handblown glass globe filled with white sand that I kept on the windowsill next to our bed. Will's mom had bought it at a museum gift shop during her last visit. The glass, streaked pink and lavender and tangerine, reminded her of the sunsets in Santa Barbara, and she had given it to me as a stand-in until I was well enough to travel and see them for myself. Palming the globe in my right hand, I admired the iridescent swirl of sand inside. Then, I lifted it high above my head and chucked it as hard as I could across the room. I'm a terrible shot and the globe missed Will by about five feet—it didn't even reach the far wall of our tiny apartment but instead plummeted and exploded on the floor, broken glass and sand flying everywhere. The floor was weirdly sparkling, as if it had been dusted with glitter. I felt a sweet, flashing release as I took in the mess, the fury in my core loosening.

"What the hell?" Will spluttered, his mouth dropping open in shock.

"This is my hell," I bawled back.

I got up from bed, shards of glass crunching beneath my slippers, and went to the bathroom, slamming the door shut. I bent over the sink and splashed my face with cold water and looked in the mirror. I looked horrible—because I was horrible, I thought, with a nauseating swell of shame. Along with the chemo, an ugliness was coursing through my veins. Small violences. Swallowed resentment. Buried humiliations. Displaced fury. And a marrow-deep weariness at a situation that had dragged on far longer than either of us could bear. These were the things that infected the growing distance between Will and me. These were the things I could talk about with Melissa, who understood better than anyone the bifurcation of personality that can happen when you're sick—how illness heightens the good and the bad, unveiling new parts of yourself you wish you hadn't known were there; how illness can bring you down to your most savage self.

But to try to explain this to Will seemed impossible. So I slipped out of the bathroom, and without a word, we got into bed. Through the thin drapes, I could see the snow still falling. I had gone too far and wished I could take back what I'd done. I tried to say *I'm sorry,* but he was already asleep.

Early the next morning Will bought a last-minute plane ticket, packed a bag, and left for Texas.

20

A MOTLEY CREW

MELISSA WAS THE most beautiful woman I had ever seen up close, and I wasn't the only one to think so. With her silver snakeskin clogs, her tattoos, and her older-woman sophistication, she quickly became the glamorous pied piper of the pediatric cancer ward. Several of the teenage boys had developed debilitating crushes on her, their cheeks reddening whenever they dragged their IV poles past.

One of them was Johnny, the same boy I had chatted with online while undergoing my transplant. He was a skinny, good-looking kid from Michigan, with an olive complexion and eyes like chocolate. His freshman year of college had been cut short by a leukemia diagnosis. Now he lived at the Ronald McDonald House, the pediatric equivalent of the Hope Lodge, where sick kids and their parents who came from far away had the option of living for next to nothing. Johnny's mother, a pious Colombian woman with a heavy accent, accompanied him everywhere he went, but when he was with Melissa and me, he would banish her to the waiting room, saying, "Mo-om, can't you see I'm trying to hang out with my friends?" Johnny had quickly developed a crush on Melissa and wanted desperately for us to think he was cool—he loved to talk about the fraternity he had briefly joined, the wild keg parties, the girls. We didn't necessarily buy his tales, which often sounded exaggerated and hard to believe, but he was earnest and sweet and we came to love him like a little brother.

Another of Melissa's fans was a young man named Max Ritvo. He was a poet, in his senior year at Yale. He split his time between his dorm room in New Haven and an apartment that his family had rented for him in a posh building with marble floors and a white-gloved elevator attendant a few blocks north of the hospital. Like most everyone else at Sloan Kettering, Max was as bald and pale as a boiled egg, but he stood out from the other patients with his thrift-store kimono, tortoiseshell spectacles, and a tattoo of a bird inked onto the side of his skull. Max, like Melissa, had Ewing sarcoma, which he'd been in treatment for on and off since the age of sixteen. He was brilliant and funny, with a brain that spouted aphorisms and metaphors so strange and vivid they made us pause mid-conversation to laugh. Max described morphine withdrawal as feeling like "a sobbing window pane having hammers and acid taken to it." Scan anxiety was like "eating a pizza and not being sure if those are pepper flakes or small red mites." Losing his virginity in a hospital bed was like "having sex on a lumpy raft in the middle of a sea of antiseptic." His phrases so perfectly encapsulated our very particular sufferings that I often found myself scribbling them on scraps of paper, tucking them into the back pocket of my jeans for safekeeping.

We formed a motley cancer crew, one that only grew as the months passed. There was Kaylin, the punk-rock fashion designer with sleeves of tattoos, who also had Ewing sarcoma and, when she couldn't find a place to live, moved into Melissa's apartment in

Brooklyn and became her roommate; Kristen, who had lymphoma and owned a small skateboard shop in the West Village; Erika, a graduate student in the Food Studies program at NYU, with breast cancer, who had a quirky sense of humor and always came to our hangs with gourmet snacks; and Anjali, an immigrant from India with my same diagnosis, who had a caustic attitude, swore constantly, and was infamous for having once made a nurse cry. I'd met Anjali in the waiting room of the outpatient bone marrow clinic. She was in her late thirties, pretty, with tawny skin and a beaked nose like mine, and always dressed in the requisite patient uniform: a knit ski cap pulled over her bald head and a face mask slapped across hollowed cheeks. The first time we saw each other, she'd nodded at me and I'd nodded back, both of us acknowledging the rare sighting: a fellow young woman in an ocean of wrinkled white faces. "So tired of looking at old farts," she'd told me, rolling her eyes at the other patients, and like that we became friends. Anjali's brother, her best potential match for a donor, had never returned her calls. Her transplant had failed.

Within the crew, we devised an unofficial buddy system. We accompanied each other to chemo and compared treatment notes. Watched soap opera marathons when we were too tired to chat and played Words with Friends when insomnia hijacked our nights. Showed up at each other's doorsteps with takeout and Xanax when someone got bad medical news. Took each other shopping when our clothing no longer fit our changing bodies and picked up the phone in the middle of the night when the anxiety attacks struck. Eventually, we would hold hospice vigils and help plan memorials. But we didn't know this yet.

Shortly after all of us started hanging out, I was invited to speak at a young adult cancer conference in Las Vegas, and I proposed we make a girls' trip out of it. Anjali wasn't well enough to come, but the rest of us—Melissa, Kaylin, Erika, Kristen, and I—had gotten the green light from our doctors, and we boarded a plane early one Friday morning, armed with face masks and a Tupperware of pot brownies.

The lobby of the Palms Resort in downtown Vegas had gaudy chandeliers, pleather couches, wall-to-wall red carpet that reeked of smoke, and dozens of slot machines. When we checked in at the front desk, the receptionist told us that we'd been upgraded—to the penthouse. Unable to believe our luck, we rode the elevator to the top floor and flung open the doors to the suite to find two huge rooms with floor-to-ceiling windows overlooking the city, all lit up and strobing with flashing billboards. In the living room was a glass shower outfitted with a stripper pole that we took turns twirling around, howling with laughter until our ribs ached. We unpacked our suitcases, and the coffee table was soon covered in wigs. On the bar, we lined up all of our medications like shot glasses; between the five of us, we had more than a hundred pill bottles.

We spent most of that day at the pool, then went to a tattoo parlor called Precious Slut. Since her diagnosis, Melissa had gotten dozens of tattoos. It was a trend I'd noticed among young cancer patients: a desire to stake a claim to your body and to take control, to make of it a canvas of your own design. In a nod to our weekend in Vegas—to the strange circumstances that had brought us together—Melissa and Kaylin got matching spades on their forearms and begged us to join them. Erika already had a tattoo, a Chinese character she'd gotten as a teenager on her lower back and now fiercely regretted, claiming that with time and gravity it had migrated halfway down her ass. Kristen wasn't an ink girl and though I was tempted, I was still too immunocompromised.

Later that night, back at the hotel, we ordered champagne and a couple of pizzas, and curled up like cats on the white couches in the living room. We talked into the wee hours about everything from post-chemo hairstyling tips and fears of relapse to the hot young chef from New Zealand whom Erika had met on an online dating site. "I wanted to get laid one more time before they lop off my boobs," said Erika, who was scheduled to have a double mastectomy in the next few weeks. She had kept her wig on during her night with the chef and hadn't told him she was sick, though she'd caught him eyeing the LIVESTRONG bracelet on her wrist once or twice. Over the next week, they'd texted back and forth, but Erika didn't know how to proceed without telling him the truth. She pulled out her phone and began reading the text she had sent him out loud: "Hi, this is probably the worst text you'll ever receive in your life, but I feel like I need to tell you, because I think you might actually like me. I have cancer and the real reason I can't see you this week is because I am doing chemotherapy. I'm so sorry. Please don't feel obligated to even respond!"

We all leaned in, breathless. "What'd he say?" Kaylin asked.

"Nothing," Erika told us. "But an hour later I heard a knock on my door. It was a bouquet delivery, these beautiful artisanal flowers from a shop on my street that I love. I opened the card and it said: 'Doesn't change a thing. XOXO, Mike.'"

"Okay, so obviously this guy is a keeper. But what we really want to know is, how was the sex?" Kristen asked.

Erika sighed. "Honestly? Best of my life."

"Jealous," I blurted out.

"But you and Will are the perfect couple," Melissa insisted. "You two are the only reason I still believe in love."

The truth of what was happening with Will—the tension and the growing distance, the frustration and resentment—was something I couldn't fully admit to myself. So instead of sharing all this with these women, to whom I could talk about almost anything, I simply shrugged.

Sex had always been a big part of my relationship with Will, even after my diagnosis. If anything, illness had intensified our passion, filling us with a weird lusty hunger for each other. We had made a careful study out of how to fuck in a hospital room without getting caught, though our tactics weren't always foolproof. (At Mount Sinai, we'd been caught more than once by the nurses who took to knocking loudly on my hospital room door and asking, "Everybody clothed?" before entering.) But things had changed in recent months.

Our first attempt at intimacy since the transplant had happened late one night while we were still at the Hope Lodge. Will had returned from a college reunion downtown and he'd climbed into my twin bed, kissing me. I had lost all bodily desire since the transplant—to eat, to move, to touch, or to be touched. My skin was raw and tender, and the steroids I was prescribed to treat the GVHD left me feeling bloated and irritable. I felt uncomfortable and nauseated all the time, and also guilty about how unavailable I'd been. That's why I didn't say no when he slid on top of me. I wanted things to be normal again—but they weren't. My brain blurred with pain. It felt like my insides were cleaving and ripping and tearing. I cried out again and again, but Will mistook my cries for pleasure and I didn't correct him. I wanted to act the part of a girlfriend; to give him this, when I had so little else left to give. Afterward, I went to the bathroom and locked the door. I sat in there for a long time, long enough that the blood coating the insides of my thighs had dried.

I couldn't understand what was happening to my body. I didn't know why my skin would suddenly burn up, hot as a kettle, making me tear off the blankets in the middle of the night and dunk my head under a faucet of cold water. I didn't know how to control my moods, which swung and swirled, making me shout from frustration one minute and leaving me euphoric the next. I didn't know why I'd suddenly tear up while I was waiting in line at the grocery store or sitting in the dog park. Since Will and I moved into the East Village apartment and started sharing a bed again, I'd become an expert in avoidance—turning my back to him at night, mumbling excuses about being too tired, or pretending to be asleep. On the rare occasions when we were intimate, I turned into the kind of woman who focuses her eyes on a crack in the ceiling and vacates her body, waiting for it to be over.

No one on my medical team had ever broached the topic of sexual health and cancer during my treatment. No one warned me that menopause is a common side effect of the treatment I had undergone. No one advised me about the available remedies to help with the hot flashes and pain. I had waited for my period to return after the transplant; it never came. At the age of twenty-four, *menopause* wasn't even a word in my vocabulary. In turn, I'd kept quiet about the changes in my body, believing that something must be wrong with me. I'd told no one about what I was experiencing—not my medical team, not Will, not my mother, not anyone—until now.

On our last evening in Vegas, my throat tightened as I began to confide in my friends. I told them about the pain that night at the Hope Lodge, and about the frustration and confusion I'd felt afterward. To my surprise, Melissa and Kaylin chimed in, saying that sex had also become painful for them and that they wondered if it was a side effect of the pelvic radiation they'd received. Kristen said that since finishing chemo, it was so excruciating, she simply couldn't do it. Erika talked about her oncologist's visible discomfort when she'd asked him about safe birth control methods. "I felt like I was having a conversation with my uncle," she told us. So, after her tryst with the chef, she'd turned to the Internet to find out if it was safe for her to take a morning-after pill.

That night, we were just a group of young women who had received little to no information about the sexual side effects of our disease, trying to puzzle it out together. I cried afterward, overcome by an odd combination of emotions: heartbreak over our shared loss and profound relief—even joy—about breaking through the silence, the shame of it all, together.

21

HOURGLASS

TIME IS BOTH slow and slippery when you're sick, when your days are consumed with the task of caring for the ever-breaking machinery of the body. Though all you want is *more* time to live, you pray for the pain meds to take effect quickly, for night to come soon, but the minutes and hours inch forward, taking their sweet damn time. Then the bigger increments of time—the weeks and months of suffering—whiz past in a blur of doctors' appointments, transfusions, and trips to the emergency room.

This paradox was especially true in the autumn of 2013. Somehow, an entire year had passed since I'd started the maintenance chemo after the transplant, and on a Friday morning, I prepared for what I thought would be my last day of treatment. I dressed up for the occasion and chose a cotton sundress with a floral print that matched my mood—airy, bright, hopeful. It showed off my tan from a recent trip with some friends to the Long Island shore, an early—if somewhat premature—celebration of the day. En route to the hospital, I sat alone in a row of blue plastic seats on the M15 express bus, content to daydream. Leaning my cheek against the glass, I studied the bustle of traffic swarming First Avenue.

When I arrived at Sloan Kettering, I was on time, for once. Seated on the exam table, legs dangling over the edge, I pulled down the strap of my dress to reveal my port, a small hockey-puck-shaped object lodged under the skin between my right collarbone and my right breast. I winced as the nurse inserted a needle into it, connecting me to the IV bag of chemo. When she flushed the line I could taste the hit of saline in the back of my throat, briny and comforting in its familiarity. Then she hung the bag on the pole and adjusted the valve on the tubing until she hit the right drip-to-minute ratio.

"How are you feeling today?" she asked. She had pink-glossed lips, a blond messy bun, and a face like a sugar cookie—pale, round, sweet.

"I can't believe this is it," I said. "Do I get to ring a bell? Or is there some kind of diploma for being done with chemo?"

The nurse squinted at me, her forehead crinkling in confusion. "Dr. Castro didn't tell you?"

"Tell me what?"

"Oh," she said. "He talked it over with the rest of the transplant team. Based on new guidelines and research, they think you should do another nine months of the chemo—just to be on the safe side."

"Another nine months?"

This was not a novel feeling: my sense of safety being demolished in the amount of time it takes to utter a sentence. *You have leukemia. The treatments are not working. You need a transplant. You need more chemo.* Words had been my salvation since I'd started writing the column, and I had almost forgotten how much they could hurt; how they could so easily destroy your plans for the future, for a life. The tears came reflexively, hot and fast, in sheets down my cheeks. "Can I talk to Dr. Castro?"

"He's not in today," replied the nurse. She handed me a box of tissues and apologized again about the mix-up. I told her not to worry. It wasn't her fault, it wasn't anyone's fault—or, if it was, it didn't matter. There was never any question that I would agree to the extra chemo—I had come this far, and I would continue doing whatever was needed to survive. "See you in three weeks," I said when the infusion was finished.

Later that night, I worked up the courage to tell Will what had happened at the hospital, then searched his face for clues to see how he was taking the news. Another nine months of doctors' appointments, medical bills, and debilitating exhaustion. Another nine months of his life being derailed by my health. We got into bed and Will murmured all the right words of support. He told me how sorry he was, that it was okay to be angry. He kissed my face and gently wiped my cheeks with his palms when the tears came again. These kindnesses meant everything, but it was difficult for me to know how he really felt. Will was as opaque as I was prone to emotional outbursts. If he was pissed off or sad or disappointed, I almost never found out until after the fact. When he fell asleep, I watched him, wondering what was happening behind those hooded, blue eyes.

A week later, Will sat me down in the living room and told me he was leaving for California. The plan was for him to take a break— a longer one this time so that he could recharge and spend time with his parents, whom he hadn't seen in a while. He would work remotely from their home in Santa Barbara. A month—maybe two, tops. Plus, I could visit, he added. Maybe we could even go on that California road trip I'd been fantasizing about. "Couples take space all the time," he said. "I think this could be really good for us."

I stared at him slack-jawed. The plan sounded so simple and straightforward when he laid it out like that—and in the alternate universe where we were a normal couple, it could have been. But that wasn't our reality. We were boyfriend and girlfriend, but also caregiver and patient. I resented him for forcing me to spell this out—for making me list all the ways in which I was dependent on him.

The list included the renovations on our apartment kitchen that were about to begin—renovations that I would suddenly be left to handle without him. The help I needed when I was sick. Walking the dog, grocery shopping, cooking, picking up prescriptions from the pharmacy, midnight trips to urgent care, and on and on. Our tiny apartment was three and a half hours away from my parents, and with no spare bedroom for them, they couldn't stay comfortably for longer than a few nights. I would have to move back into my childhood bedroom in Saratoga while Will was gone—something I had no desire to do—or to manage here on my own.

"Are you leaving because I have to do more chemo?" I asked.

"Of course not," he snapped. "How could you say that? I've sacrificed everything for you."

Immediately I felt guilty. He was right about the sacrifices, of course, but still, I wanted to know: "Then why are you leaving?"

"I need to focus on myself. I'm not happy, and I'm not where I want to be professionally. I spend all day editing other people's work, helping them make *their* dreams come true, and then I come home and I take care of you."

"But why can't you work on yourself here?" I said. "I can help."

"Between your cancer treatment and your career, you take up a lot of space in this relationship."

There was truth to Will's words. Over the last year, the popularity of the column had led to magazine profiles and television appearances, followed by some speaking engagements. In a surreal twist, I'd even won a News & Documentary Emmy Award for the video series that accompanied the column. Attending the glitzy ceremony at Lincoln Center, I felt equally excited and out of place, with my cheeks swollen from the steroids and my hair in a quarter-inch crop. Each time an opportunity had appeared, I had said yes, wanting to seize the momentum while it was there, while I could. But raw willpower and ambition can only carry you so far. I was folding under the workload and everyone in my life—my family and friends, Will, my doctors—was worried about the toll it took on my health.

From day one, Will had offered his support, and I'd grate-fully—in retrospect, too eagerly—accepted it. He'd pulled count-less all-nighters to read and to revise drafts, helped me negotiate contracts, and prepped me for interviews. The first time I was in-vited to deliver a keynote at a medical conference in Atlanta, he used his vacation days to come with me, since I was still too sick to travel alone. He pushed my wheelchair through airport security lines, carried our bags, and took care of me when I caught a virus on the plane. The added income had allowed us to live more com-fortably, and I split what I earned with him, insisting that he de-served to be compensated since there was no way I could have done any of it without him. But what had begun as a labor of love had also just become a whole lot of labor. In recent weeks, I'd tried making myself smaller, asking for less, saying less, and encourag-ing him to focus on his own creative projects, but it didn't seem to matter. I couldn't help feeling like I was always using up too much oxygen in the room. Until now, I had never heard Will confirm this out loud.

"Your unhappiness? Your professional disappointments? Those are my fault?" I asked. My hands were starting to tremble. I grabbed the prescription bottle of Xanax on the kitchen counter and crunched a couple of the baby-blue pills between my molars; they worked faster if you chewed them up rather than swallowed them whole. I wanted to avoid another eruption like the one with the glass globe, but it was too late. "Fuck you," I said in a low hiss. "Fuck you for making me feel like more of a burden than I already do."

To be a patient is to relinquish control—to your medical team and their decisions, to your body and its unscheduled breakdowns. Caregivers, by proxy, suffer a similar fate. But there are crucial differences between the two. More than ever, I wanted to walk away: from the changing treatment protocols and timelines, the exhaustion and the humiliation of having to ask for constant help. But as a sick person, I was bound to the mess of it all, to this wretched marrow of mine. As a caregiver, Will had been there out of love and also, perhaps, from a sense of obligation. The continuous refrains of "You're a saint for sticking by her—a good man, a model partner," surely did not lessen the pressure he must have felt. But being here, enduring this with me, was a choice. The truth was that he could leave. And he would.

Everyone did their best to support me when Will went to California that fall. My friends made a renewed effort to reach out and to drop off home-cooked meals from time to time, a neighbor volunteered to walk Oscar during chemo week, and my parents found someone to help clean the apartment. Will did his best from afar, calling several times a day to check up on me. For the most part, our conversations were full of the usual warmth and humor, but there were moments, especially when I was back in the emergency room or flailing under the stress of having to manage on my own, when it was hard to keep the resentment from creeping into my voice. But mostly, I just missed him. I thought often of Will's words from that first night in Saratoga after my diagnosis: *A lot of bad things are about to happen. We need to put our relationship into a box and to protect it with everything we have.* And at first we had, the illness bringing us together, closer than ever before. But somewhere along the way, both of us had stopped protecting our relationship—worse, we'd turned against it, against each other in moments. Now the illness had pushed us three thousand miles apart.

In Will's absence, I began spending more time with the cancer crew. Without my ever having to ask for anything or explain, they understood I was in a low-down place. Erika made sweatshirts with the words TEAM SUSU printed across the front in varsity letter- ing, and Kristen accompanied me to urgent care or to my chemo appointments so that I wouldn't have to be alone. Max was always showing up at my apartment with ninety-nine-cent slices of pizza and expertly rolled joints, and Melissa rallied the troops, organiz- ing game nights, dance parties, and the occasional outing. A hic- cup of genetics had brought us together—all of us bound by rogue, malignant cells and a heightened sense of our mortality— but at some point we'd become more than circumstantial friends. We were family.

One chilly evening later that fall, Melissa and I set out to meet Johnny at the Ronald McDonald House on Seventy-third Street and First Avenue. It was snowing a little, and we shivered as we stepped under the red awning and into the revolving doors. Johnny was waiting for us inside, dressed in a black suit, loose on his dis- appearing frame, and a large red tie that lapped down the front of a white dress shirt. His latest rounds of chemo had turned his skin a waxen, yellowish hue. I remember thinking how much frailer he seemed since we'd celebrated his twenty-first birthday just a few weeks earlier. Sick as he was, he had scrubbed up like a stud—and for good reason.

The Make-A-Wish Foundation is in the business of granting sick kids and teenagers a wish of their choice. I'd heard of wish recipients traveling to Spain to see matadors in bejeweled vests wave their crimson flags at testosterone-fueled bulls. Some went to Disney World to ride roller coasters with their favorite celebrities. Others requested beach vacations with their families at Hawaiian resorts. Johnny's wish, by contrast, was simple. He wanted to take the cancer crew to a nice dinner and a Broadway show, but I suspected I had been invited as a foil. Going solo on a date with Melissa would have made his crush on her too obvious.

Johnny's mom was there as usual, and his dad had flown in from Michigan for the week. They snapped dozens of pictures of the three of us as we posed in the lobby. Melissa and I stood on either side of Johnny with our arms looped through his, all of us grinning at the camera like we were headed to prom. A black limousine waited for us at the curb. The driver, dressed in a black sweater vest and a formal chauffeur cap, opened the door with a flourish. "After you," Johnny said, stepping aside so that Melissa and I could climb in first. "Ooh la la! So chivalrous," we teased as his ears turned bright pink.

The limo shimmied down Midtown's crowded streets, passing Technicolor skyscrapers and mobs of tourists. We pulled up to a building with an enormous sign out front that said: WELCOME TO FLAVORTOWN. We had arrived at Guy Fieri's eponymous restaurant in Times Square. A maître d' escorted us through a maze of tobacco-hued wood-paneled rooms to our table. Johnny was visibly excited as he opened the giant menu, reading off the items he'd been wanting to try ever since he'd first read about the restaurant—specifically, the Bacon Mac 'n' Cheese Burger and something called Awesome Pretzel Chicken Tenders. "Isn't this amazing? We can order anything and the best part is—it's all FREE!"

It made me happy to see him in such good spirits. He'd had such a rough go of things as of late. As an only child of mixed race, he hadn't been able to find a donor match. The alternative for patients in his situation was a cord blood transplant, which required him to be in full remission before starting the procedure. But each time he got close to achieving remission, a barrage of infections and complications would set him back. Recently, his leukemia had stopped responding to the treatments altogether. Now the plan was for him to travel down to MD Anderson, the big cancer hospital in Houston, where he hoped to be eligible for a new clinical trial. He was leaving in a couple of days.

We ordered champagne and toasted to the success of Johnny's upcoming clinical trial, to our crew, to better days, to Guy Fieri's terrible taste in . . . everything. Half a dozen dishes arrived, covering every inch of the big lacquered table. Johnny took a few bites, but left most of the food untouched. As dinner went on, he got quieter and quieter. By the time the dessert arrived—a deep-fried "boulder" of ice cream—he looked shaky and pale, his forehead coated in a thin film of sweat.

"You feeling all right?" I asked.

"I'm good—no, I'm better than good. This has been one of the best nights of my life and it's not even over. We still get to see a Broadway show!" he said with forced cheer.

When we arrived at the theater, the lobby was packed, and as we made our way through the crowd of shoving bodies, Johnny swayed unsteadily on his feet. We asked again if he was feeling okay, but he brushed us off, insisting he was fine. But as he walked up the carpeted steps toward the main floor of the theater, he stopped several times, leaning heavily against the banister. Melissa and I exchanged worried glances and walked discreetly behind him with our arms outstretched, ready to catch him in case he collapsed.

We made it to our section without incident, but when we showed our tickets to the usher, there was a brief, awkward moment as we realized only two of the seats were located together. Johnny looked a little uncomfortable, then mentioned that the tickets had been arranged last minute.

"So, who wants to sit where?" the usher butted in.

"Melissa," Johnny asked shyly, "wanna sit with me?"

The usher guided Melissa and Johnny to their seats, which were located a row down and to the right of mine. Soon after, the show started, lights dimming, heavy velvet curtains parting to the thrum of music. But I couldn't focus on the show. Instead, I leaned over in my seat, sneaking a glance at Johnny, checking to make sure he was all right. When I saw the ecstatic grin plastered across his face, I found myself chuckling, overcome with both pride and tenderness. Sitting next to the coolest, most beautiful girl of them all, he was better than all right.

Afterward, Melissa and I dropped Johnny off at the Ronald McDonald House. As we said goodbye, we knew there was a chance we might not see him again. I think he knew it, too. "Love you guys," he said in an uncharacteristically earnest display of affection, then wrapped us into a gruff hug.

Three weeks later, Johnny's mother called me from Texas. "Pneumonia, cardiac arrest"—her words came out in splintered sobs. "We don't know nobody here. I need to get my boy home." It was hard to make out what was happening. Then: "Johnny boy is with God now."

22

THE EDGES OF US

WHEN WILL CAME home from California just after Christmas, I don't know who was more relieved, me or the dog. I think it might have been Oscar, given that he peed all over the rug in excitement when Will walked through the door. In his absence, I'd realized some things. One was that I had been working and writing like I was running out of time, and I'd been running myself and our relationship ragged in the process. I also realized I couldn't imagine life without Will and that I didn't want to. The final thing I understood was that if something didn't change soon, the damage to our relationship would be beyond repair.

Eager for quality time together, I suggested we head up to Saratoga. Since my parents were traveling, we'd have the house to ourselves. We packed a suitcase and the three of us boarded a train. We woke up the next morning to a foot of fresh snow, everything twinkling and untainted. Will and I wrapped ourselves up like mummies in hats and scarves, donned bulky coats and boots, and headed outdoors. Will began shoveling the driveway as Oscar raced through the snow in frenzied circles. I watched for a while, then gathered some snow in my mittens, pressed it into a ball and threw it at Will—resulting in a full-scale, exhilarating snowball fight. "I feel like Kevin McCallister in *Home Alone!*" I shouted, pinning him in the back of the head.

We passed the next few days this way, indulging in each other's company, enjoying our little escape. Then on New Year's Eve, we drove to a friend's party in the nearby town of Millbrook. As Will steered the minivan down a frozen highway, we chatted about our resolutions. That year, there was an added sense of importance to the ritual, an urgency to get things right. We both agreed that we needed help and decided to look into couples therapy. We also talked about finding a change of scenery. Both of us were desperate to get out of the city, which had become synonymous with hospitals and heartbreak. We fantasized about moving into a little farmhouse in the Hudson Valley, somewhere quiet with a big backyard where Oscar could run free and we could plant a garden— where we could start over again. Or maybe we'd buy a car and live on the road for a while, exploring the country and camping in national parks until we found a new place to call home. "Let's promise to lean on each other during these next months. We can't let all that's happened push us apart," Will said. "The harder things are, the closer we should be. It's our job. The most important job. I love you."

It was everything I'd been wanting and needing to hear, and by the time we arrived at the party, I was glowing. In the hours that followed, we made good on the old edict—we ate, drank, and were merry. Our host took out a guitar and everyone sang along to Beatles songs. I sat on Will's lap, our bodies swaying together to the music. Lizzie was there and at one point she pulled me aside. "I love seeing you and Will looking so happy," she said. "I haven't seen you like this in a long time." She then told me that she and a handful of my closest friends had recently gotten an email from Will. In essence, he'd written that, although he wanted to respect my privacy, he also thought they needed to know the toll that my ongoing treatment had been taking on both of us. He wondered if they might be available as extra reinforcements, especially the weeks during and right after chemo, when the side effects were the worst. Will suggested creating an email chain, so that when he was working or couldn't be home at night, someone else might be able to step in to help. Ending on an upbeat, he thanked everyone for their support: *Most of all, I want to say if I haven't in a while that I love you all and I'm so happy you're looking out for Suleika. She doesn't always let on how hard things are . . . But she's strong, as we know.* That Will had taken such a step made me feel both annoyed—that he hadn't consulted me—and hopeful. It showed he was taking our problems seriously, that he was already looking for ways to make things better.

As midnight approached, someone suggested we go ice-skating. Everyone grabbed a bottle of champagne and a pair of skates, and we trekked through the snow toward the lake way out on the edge of the property. Will took my mittened hands in his as we skittered onto the ice. Everyone counted down to 2014, shouting at the moon. "To a better year," I said, pulling him close. "To a better year," he repeated, and we kissed.

When we returned to the city, we made good on our resolution to start couples therapy. We found our first therapist through the yellow pages. Her office had a ratty couch and a threadbare Persian rug. The air reeked of patchouli. She seemed ill-versed in the nuances of navigating a relationship during a long illness and she didn't take insurance, so after a couple of unhelpful sessions we decided to move on. The second therapist we saw was part of the psycho-oncology program at Sloan Kettering and was covered by my insurance. Dr. T was kind and a good listener, but most of the time we left her office angrier about what had been said and heavier for what we'd learned of each other, feeling more rudderless than ever.

One day, Dr. T asked us if we might be willing to have one of our sessions observed by a group of residents. I agreed right away. Sloan Kettering was a teaching hospital, and I was always open to letting medical students observe. It seemed like a small sacrifice if our misfortunes could help someone else down the line. And I thought it might be helpful to hear other perspectives. But the session was a disaster. Will and I sat with Dr. T in the middle of a large conference room, as a row of strangers stood against the wall, observing us and jotting down notes on little pads of paper. It was humiliating to discuss the most painful and personal details of our relationship in front of spectators, and to have these details dissected into teaching moments.

"Most of the young, unmarried couples we see who go through extended cancer treatment together end up splitting up," one of the residents informed us. "What would help you at this stage?"

"If we knew, we wouldn't be here," Will said, in a rare, open display of anger, the tendons in his neck twitching.

A dark cloud hovered over us as we left the appointment. "We're never going back there again," we both agreed. But we desperately needed guidance. Neither of us knew how to keep going, separately or together, anymore. And yet, the more guidance we received, the more defeated we felt.

Our friends and family would have been surprised to learn we were in such a bad place, as Will and I never fought or bickered publicly. In fact, it was the opposite—in front of others, it was all awe and affection. He marveled at me and I marveled at him, and we touched almost constantly, sitting shoulder to shoulder or holding hands. He was always doting on me—snapping photographs of me and bringing me glasses of water and tucking a blanket around my legs, or explaining my absence when I had to cancel plans to rest. We finished each other's sentences without realizing it, and we were bound by a shared history that no one else could understand. Our loyalty to each other was oceanic.

In the privacy of our apartment, however, we had the same screaming arguments night after night. *Why are you so distant,* went my song. *I need a break,* went his. Oscar took to hiding under the couch until our voices returned to normal decibels. I started popping small handfuls of Xanax each time I knew we were on the verge of a big fight. Sometimes, I'd reflexively take one as soon as I heard his keys jangling in the front door. My anger was slowly being replaced by a muted resignation. Any hints of intimacy, sexual or otherwise, were gone. Come bedtime, we'd switch off the lights and lie back to back, silently stewing, preferring to commune with our phones instead of each other.

Will had to return to work and as we said goodbye, I felt overwhelmed with a sense of something looming. I hugged him longer than usual, not wanting to let go, a lump of fear forming in my throat. It was the fear of loving someone whom you can't bear to lose. Of knowing that the end might be near.

As I took the bus home that day, I reminded myself that Will was still here, by my side, after almost three years of treatment. I tried to convince myself that our relationship could still be resuscitated. I wanted to believe that it was simply a question of putting in more work, of trying harder and seeking out better help. *Cancer is greedy,* I thought. *It has ravaged not only my body, but every single thing I've believed to be true about myself, and now it has metastasized to our relationship, ruining what was good and pure between us.*

I wished more than anything that I could travel back in time. I would have been more vigilant about protecting our love. I would have started couples therapy on the day I was diagnosed. I would have refused to let Will sleep next to my hospital bed night after night and I would have leaned more on my parents. I would have tried harder to process the anger that, with no release valve, had welled and pressurized in me over time. But there was no turning back the hands of the clock and the way forward was unclear. The solution to our problems seemed beyond reach: a boat, lost in the fog, drifting farther and farther away.

23

THE LAST GOOD NIGHT

TO THE POLICE officer, we must have looked like two more tough girls with terrible attitudes. We were decked out in matching black leather jackets. I was sporting a fresh buzz cut and heavy eyeliner, and a large tattoo of a python glistened on my neck. Melissa's hair spilled to her waist, a dozen silver rings adorned her fingers, and her pupils were dilated from the pot she smoked almost hourly these days.

What the police officer couldn't have known was that my neck tattoo was fake, that Melissa was wearing a wig, and that she had recently learned that her Ewing sarcoma was terminal. Earlier that week the doctors had told her there was nothing more they could do for her. She had started exploring clinical options, shopping for time, but the prognosis was grim. To cheer her up, I'd proposed a night out on the town. So we'd made our way to a motorcycle and tattoo festival, then danced on our chairs under the sparkling lights of a disco ball at a drag burlesque show. And now we were here—standing face-to-face with a cop on a subway platform in Coney Island, the first hints of dawn seeping into the night.

A few minutes earlier, we'd jumped the turnstile, even though both of us had MetroCards in our wallets. When facing death, the phrase YOLO—you only live once—takes on new meaning. But we had broken the law, the police officer said, and he threatened to haul us down to the local precinct. Without missing a beat, Melissa pulled off her wig, revealing her bald scalp. Her eyes glossed over with tears as she launched into an impressive fib about being in a rush to get home so that she could take her cancer meds. Her performance worked, and the cop let us off easy, issuing us two hundred-dollar tickets. He even apologized for having to give us tickets at all, but said that since we'd been caught on camera, he didn't have a choice.

"Partners in crime," Melissa said to me under her breath after the cop wished us well and sent us on our way.

"Bad to the bone—literally diseased," I quipped back. The second we got on the subway and the doors closed behind us, we fell over each other, shrieking with laughter.

It was the last good night we'd have together, but we didn't know it. One rarely does.

Eight weeks later, on a Monday morning in early March, I went to Sloan Kettering for my second-to-last cycle of chemo, but instead of feeling relief that I was almost done, my thoughts kept turning to Melissa. Her cancer was spreading through her body with terrifying speed and the tumors were ruthless. They had fractured her spine in two places and were pushing through her skull, distorting her delicate features and swelling one of her eyes shut. Melissa said she felt ugly and didn't want anyone to see her. With the exception of me, Max, and a few of her closest friends, she refused all visitors.

When people imagine dying, they seem to gravitate toward certain stories. In eulogies and obituaries, they invoke phrases like *passed away, being called home,* or *gained her angel wings.* These euphemisms make death sound so passive and peaceful, like drifting off into a midday nap. They prefer to think that when the time comes, a person feels somehow prepared. That was not the case with Melissa. She raged as death grew more imminent. "I'm not ready," she'd say. "I still have so much to do." She was also terrified, obsessing over what it would be like—and how her parents would cope.

Every day that week, after I finished up my infusion, I rode the elevator to the eighteenth floor, where she was an inpatient. Each time I showed up she seemed sicker and sicker. One day, before entering her room, I saw her parents in the hallway. "The doctors keep telling us to prepare ourselves, we need to prepare ourselves," her father said, rubbing his puffy eyes with balled fists, as if trying to wake from a nightmare.

When I went to see Melissa another day, she asked me if I wanted to go on a trip with her back to India. She thought we should leave right away. "I don't have much time," she slurred, her voice soaked with morphine. I sat quietly for a moment, searching for the right words to respond. Over the last few years I'd watched my friends and family force upbeat smiles and blink back tears as they sat by my own hospital bed. Now, as I struggled to do the same, I stared up at the ceiling and swallowed hard, then bit my bottom lip as I tried to keep my composure.

"Where should we travel to first?" I asked.

There was no way Melissa could board a flight to anywhere. But we planned an itinerary anyway, imagining a trip that we both knew would never come to pass: the rickshaws we would ride through downtown Delhi, all the hand-painted marionettes we would buy at the market to add to her collection, a visit to the Taj Mahal at sunrise. I smiled brightly, nodding as she spoke, jumping in here and there with suggestions and murmurs of encouragement. India had become a metaphor rather than a destination.

As Melissa began nodding off, I got up to leave. I squeezed her hand and stooped down to give her a hug. "I'm not ready," she said tearfully. I tucked her in, pulling up the white hospital blanket and drawing the blinds. "Get some rest," I said softly. "I'll be back to see you tomorrow." I paused in the doorway, just a moment, to watch her sleep.

The next morning, Melissa was loaded into an ambulance and transferred to a hospice center in Massachusetts so she could be closer to home. She posted a photograph to Instagram, taken from inside the ambulance, two frosted windows looking out onto a busy avenue. "Bye New York. I loved you. My heart is broken," she wrote in the caption below.

I didn't get to see her before she left. At the same moment that her ambulance pulled away, I was tied to an IV pole, a last bag of poison dripping into my veins.

Death never comes at a good time, but getting a death sentence when you're young is a breach of contract with the natural order of things. After years of being sick, Melissa and I had learned to coexist with the threat of death as best we could. Mortality was a stench we couldn't wash off, no matter how hard we tried. We talked about it at length. Sometimes, we even joked about it. Melissa said she wanted everyone to cry a lot at her funeral. I said I wanted mine to have a raucous after-party, and together we drew up a rider, detailing the guest list and what kind of cocktails would be served.

But nothing could have prepared me for actually losing her. The sheer number of times we had flirted with death and then recovered had, in a strange way, made us feel invincible. Even after Melissa left New York; even after she stopped answering text messages, her mind traveling to the watery space between the living and that other place; even after her parents wrote to say that in her final hours she was surrounded by family and dozens of doodads and trinkets and those hand-painted marionettes—it didn't compute. It still doesn't compute.

The friend I could unapologetically talk to about everything was gone. But gone where?

And why?

Grief is a ghost that visits without warning. It comes in the night and rips you from your sleep. It fills your chest with shards of glass. It interrupts you mid-laugh when you're at a party, chastising you that, just for a moment, you've forgotten. It haunts you until it becomes a part of you, shadowing you breath for breath.

24

DONE

ON MY LAST day of chemo, my friends and family congratulated me on finally being "done." After countless biopsies, antibiotic drips, and vomit buckets I was supposed to be rejoining the greater gathering. But in fact, the hardest part of my cancer treatment began once it was over.

In the next month, I was hospitalized four times for a life-threatening *C. diff* intestinal infection I caught as a result of my weakened immune system. I nicknamed this month the "carnival of horrors" because each of the hospitalizations brought with it a relentless procession of surreal, harrowing events, breaking me piece by piece until there was nothing left of me to break.

The night before the first hospitalization, Melissa died.

During the second hospitalization, Erika and the chef got married in a small ceremony in Colorado, but instead of being her bridesmaid, as I'd promised, I was tethered to an IV pole.

A few days before the third hospitalization, Will began talking about taking a more drastic kind of break. He said he was thinking about moving out of our apartment and into one of his own. The idea was for us to live separately but still be together. He framed it as temporary, but I wasn't buying it.

Will's proposition hit me like a shiv to the back. A part of me had been bracing for this moment for a long time, but still I found myself reeling. It seemed unforgivable that he would do this to me now, when I was raw from Melissa's death and an infection was ravaging my guts. I wondered if this was his way of baby-stepping toward a permanent breakup. Even if, as he claimed, this was just a temporary arrangement and he eventually moved back in, I didn't see how it would help us solve anything.

I had always believed in a world where love could overcome anything. I believed love could redeem suffering and transform the brutality of a life into something bearable, even beautiful. But I was losing trust that the next time things got hard, he wouldn't up and leave again. I was losing faith in us.

I threw one last Hail Mary pass and did what the desperate do: I issued Will an ultimatum. "Either you stay and we figure out how to get through this together, or you move out and we are done," I said. "I can't keep doing this."

Twenty-four hours later Will found an apartment in Brooklyn with a move-in date scheduled for two weeks away. When he told me he was considering renting it, I did nothing to stop him. Rather, I pushed him away. "Go, what do I care?" I said, though every inch of me wanted to scream the opposite. Before I could fully process what was happening, Will signed the lease and I was back in the emergency room with another *C. diff* attack.

It was my fourth and final hospital stay. I was admitted to the eighteenth floor and placed in a room next door to where I had last seen Melissa. It felt like a cruel joke that, out of the hundreds of hospital rooms at Sloan Kettering, I would end up here. Melissa and I even had the same nurse, a woman named Maureen with a fire-hydrant-red pixie and matching lipstick. I begged to be transferred to the leukemia or transplant floor, but the hospital was over capacity, so there was nothing anyone could do. Being forced to sleep just a few feet away from where I had said goodbye to my dead best friend felt personal—a punishment intended to push me over the edge.

The day I was discharged from the hospital was the day Will moved out. When I arrived home, toting a large plastic bag from the hospital labeled PATIENT THINGS, the apartment was quiet, eerily so. *You should cry,* I told myself as I stood in the doorway, but I was too tired to cry. I wandered around the apartment, a confused Oscar trailing behind me, as I inspected the empty closets and dresser drawers with a strange methodical finality. In one of the drawers I discovered an old pack of cigarettes. I knew better, but I lit one up anyway. I sat on the kitchen floor and smoked it slowly, my hospital bracelet still wrapped around my wrist.

The inner scaffolding that had been supporting me since my diagnosis had crumbled. While in treatment, I had been surrounded by the world's best cavalry: my boyfriend, my family and friends, and a brilliant medical team that had worked tirelessly to keep me alive. The goal had been to get rid of the cancer. But now that I was done with the "cut, poison, burn" part of the disease, I sat dazed and alone in the rubble, unsure how to move on, wondering where everyone had gone and what to do from here.

I hadn't noticed the fine print until now: When you survive something that was thought to be unsurvivable, the obvious is gained. You have your life—you have time. But it's only when you get there that you realize your survival has come at a cost.

It would take me a while to pick myself up from that kitchen floor—a lost year spent seething and grieving and struggling to find my way forward—and on that terrible day, all I could do was finish my cigarette, close the blinds, and crawl into bed. *Melissa is gone. Will is gone. My cancer is gone.* I repeated these facts to my-self, willing them to sink in, willing them to feel real, but instead, I felt only numbness. It was as if the sentient parts of me had been put under anesthesia. I couldn't tell you what I did the rest of that day, or the next, or the one after. I imagine I walked the dog, stocked up on coffee and milk, and answered the phone calls of my parents often enough that they didn't show up on my doorstep, but I can't say for sure. I was going through the motions, but in fact, I was barely there.

The only thing that pierced the numbness was the specter of Will. He'd left, but not entirely. I could feel his presence—or rather, his absence—like a phantom limb. Will had been my caregiver, my confidant, my lover, my social buffer, my best friend. At times, he'd been my literal crutch, helping me walk, feed, and bathe myself when I didn't have the strength to do so on my own. He had been too many things for one person to be for another, but I couldn't fully see this yet—only that, without Will by my side, I had no idea how to navigate the world alone.

Although I'd promised myself not to call him, the urge was never far from my mind. A week after he moved out, I caved. "Can you come over?" I said to him one night when I could no longer bear the quiet of the apartment. An hour later I heard his keys in the door. He opened it without knocking, as though we still lived there together. For a few minutes we pretended nothing had changed and he rolled around on the floor roughhousing with Oscar as he always did before standing up to hug me. Then we ordered takeout from Lil' Frankie's around the corner and made attempts at civil chitchat before things, inevitably, devolved.

This became our routine, days of silence punctuated by late-night visits, which always culminated in one of two ways: Either we'd get into a screaming fight over who had done what to land us in the mess of the present, or Will would spend the night. We never had sex—that hadn't happened in months—but I was terrified of sleeping alone, and it brought me comfort to know that he still wanted to stay over. I kept hoping that being together like this, curled up with the dog like old times, would make Will realize what he was risking and that he'd apologize and move back in for good. But our togetherness, what was left of it, felt hollow. Each time, when morning came and he got up to leave, I felt humiliated and hurt. *Never again,* I vowed as I locked the door behind him, promising myself to stop calling, to stop inviting him over.

Alone in the apartment once again, I alternated between hating Will in a fervent, venomous way and lying dazed on the kitchen floor. In my mind, I was rewriting our life together as a simplistic screenplay, and the story arc went something like this: *I got sick and Will got sick of my sickness, slowly distancing himself over time until he abruptly moved out, abandoning me while I was in the hospital.* It was easier for me to frame it this way, to put all the blame on Will, than to reckon with the other parts of the story: all the ways in which I'd failed him, driving him to burnout—driving him to leave. The deeper truth of why we ended smoldered beneath the surface, still too hot to probe.

Will was my great love—I was pretty sure that this would always be the case—but as much as I wanted to think that with enough time and space we would eventually find our way back together, I no longer believed this was possible. We'd been mired in the caregiver-patient dynamic for so long that our resentment had hardened around us, trapping us like flies in amber. To keep waiting for Will was to invite the probability of more grief, more pain, more fury, and that I didn't think I could bear. For the first time in my life I had the distinct feeling of having reached a precipice that I hadn't known was there until I was teetering on the edge. I'd reached the limit of what I could endure.

The way I was beginning to see it, I had a choice to make: If I wanted a shot at finding my place among the living, I would need to stop fighting for a relationship that had flatlined long ago. I would need to start fighting for myself.

PART
TWO

25

THE IN-BETWEEN PLACE

"EVERYONE WHO IS born holds dual citizenship, in the kingdom of the well and in the kingdom of the sick," Susan Sontag wrote in *Illness as Metaphor.* "Although we all prefer to use only the good passport, sooner or later each of us is obliged, at least for a spell, to identify ourselves as citizens of that other place."

By the time I reached my last day of chemo, I'd spent the majority of my adult life in that other realm: the kingdom of the sick no one cares to inhabit. Initially, I'd clung to the hope of a short sojourn, one in which I wouldn't have to unpack my bags. I'd resisted the label of "cancer patient," believing I could remain the person I'd been. But as I grew sicker, I'd watched my old self vanish. In place of my name, I had been issued a patient ID number. I'd learned to speak fluent medicalese. Even my molecular identity had morphed: When my brother's stem cells engrafted in my marrow, my DNA had irreversibly mutated. With my bald head, pallor, and port, illness became the first thing that people noticed about me. As months bled into years, I'd adapted to the mores of this new land as best I could, befriended its inhabitants, even carved out a career within its confines. In its terrain, I'd built a home, accepting not only that I might stay there for a while, but that likely I would never leave. It was the outside world, the kingdom of the well, that had grown alien and frightening.

But for me, for all patients, the end goal is eventually to leave the kingdom of the sick. In many cancer wards, there's a bell that patients ring on their last day of treatment, a ceremonial tolling that signals a transition. It's time to say goodbye to the eerie and changeless fluorescence of hospital rooms. It's time to step back into sunlight.

It is where I find myself now, on the threshold between an old familiar state and an unknown future. Cancer no longer lives in my blood, but it lives on in other ways, dominating my identity, my relationships, my work, and my thoughts. I'm done with chemo but I still have my port, which my doctors are waiting to remove until I'm "further out of the woods." I'm left with the question of how to repatriate myself to the kingdom of the well, and whether I ever fully can. No treatment protocols or discharge instructions can guide this part of my trajectory. The way forward is going to have to be my own.

My first, inadvisable stage of recovery: immolation. I want to torch what still binds me to Will. I want to cauterize my grief. I want to burn down my past and to clear land for new growth. This, I think, is how I will start anew.

To rid the apartment of Will's ghost, I light bushels of sage. Thick scarves of smoke swirl through the air. I rearrange furniture until old rooms feel new. I collect the framed photographs of us and hide them in the dresser. I stuff the comforter we purchased down the trash chute. When he calls me, I don't reply. I delete his number.

I want so badly to be a normal twenty-six-year-old. I have no idea of what that entails, so I look to healthy peers for cues. A little less than a month after Will moves out, my friend Stacie, a singer, invites me to hear her perform at the swanky NoMad Hotel. No part of me feels up to socializing, but I force myself to go anyway. I change out of my sweatpants and T-shirt and into a dress—a hip black dress with a high neckline that conceals my port. I fuss with my hair, trying to make it look a bit less post-chemo, more punk-pixie. At the last minute, I invite an old friend to join me, one who knew me long before my sickness. He's a jazz musician named Jon.

When I arrive at the hotel, Jon is waiting in the lobby. The two of us go way back to band camp, where we met as teenagers. Jon was gangly and awkward then, with a mouth full of braces and baggy, ill-fitting clothes, so shy he bordered on mute. He's since undergone a transformation. Now, with his thick New Orleanian drawl, virtuosic piano chops, and dapper style, he has the kind of magnetic presence that turns heads and draws everyone in a room. Tall and slim, dressed impeccably in a tailored suit and leather boots, he's handsome enough to startle me. His skin, a dark honey-brown, looks luminous, and his features—those lips, aquiline nose, and broad shoulders—give him the majestic air of a prince. Jon catches my eye from across the lobby, and as I walk across the room to greet him, I wobble a little under his gaze.

We take the elevator to the second floor and enter a small, cabaret-style club with ornate wallpaper and candlelit tables, and soon Stacie ascends the stage in a red gown. As she croons into the mic, her voice seductively envelops the darkened room. Jon and I are sitting off to the side, on a plush leather couch. It's been more than a year since we last saw each other, and we have a lot to catch up on. Right away Jon asks about my health and then about Will. When I say that we are no longer together, Jon appears stunned. "Y'all seemed so . . . solid," he says.

"It's for the best," I say with contrived nonchalance, ignoring the last four weeks spent on my kitchen floor.

"What happened?" he asks. He seems genuinely perplexed.

"The illness took a toll on our relationship," I say. If I'm going to pick a perpetrator, illness is the easiest one to frame.

It's the first time I've had to explain any of this out loud. I make it sound as if it's all firmly in the past, as if it needs no untangling. I want to believe this—that moving on from my relationship with Will is going to help me move on from my illness.

"What about you?" I say, eager to change the topic. "Seeing anyone?"

"Also single," he replies.

I haven't thought of myself this way yet, as "single." Though it's technically true, I still feel in limbo. *Single.* I mouth it silently. The word feels strange on my tongue.

From the look on Jon's face it's also the first time he's considered me in this light. There's something happening between us, the air around us charged with possibility. We move on to other topics, but our conversation has taken on an edge and Jon seems to have suddenly reverted to his shy, gawky teenage self. "What's your favorite sport?" he asks out of nowhere, rocking nervously back and forth on the couch.

"My favorite *sport*?" I ask. I pause for a moment, then say the first thing that pops into my head: "Basketball, I guess."

"Wow, me too! That's another thing we have in common!" Jon says so earnestly that I can't help but laugh.

Although I've known Jon for half my life, it feels as if we are on a blind date. It is awkward. Incredibly so. I wave down the waiter and order a cocktail; when it arrives, I take long swigs. As the evening progresses, I relax a bit, and Jon seems to recover from his shyness. The music turns from jazz to a thumping bass drum, and soon everyone is talking and laughing and getting up to dance. Stacie joins us, as do a handful of girlfriends. They keep elbowing me when Jon's not looking, egging me on and telling me how it's time to start putting myself "out there" again. For the first time since leaving the hospital, I'm feeling somewhat human, even attractive.

It's well past midnight, the latest I've been out in ages, but I don't want the night to end. I want this feeling to follow me home—I *need* this feeling to follow me. Jon and I linger on the sidewalk. When he kisses my cheek good night, I feel a jolt. Deep inside, some part of me knows I'm in no place to be entertaining the idea of anything more than friendship. It's a brief moment of awareness about the state of affairs: *My personal life is a mess. My body is a mess. I am a mess.* My illness has left so much collateral damage in its wake. But to acknowledge that wreckage is to have to contend with it, and I don't feel strong enough—not yet, not anytime soon. Then the awareness passes, and I am on the other side of it. *Maybe things aren't so bad. Maybe seeing other people is part of moving on.* My mind will do anything to avoid a reckoning—it confuses and contradicts itself until I can no longer distinguish what is real from what is not; it convinces me that I'm fine when in fact I couldn't be further from it.

It isn't long before Jon and I are talking nearly every night on the phone, for hours at a stretch. He's on the road with his band, but when he returns to the city a few weeks later, he asks me out on a real date to a comedy show and dinner. Afterward, he walks me home and kisses me—this time, on the mouth. The prospect of starting a new life seems much less terrifying with someone else by my side.

I like everything about Jon. I like how his brain froths with a million ideas and his fingers stampede across the piano keys. I like his galactic ambition, which makes me want to expand the scope of my own. I like that he maintains his limitless drive without caffeine, his equilibrium without alcohol, his sanity without substances. But more than anything, I like the way I feel when I'm around him. Jon treats me like a healthy, normal, capable person—like the wild-maned, mischievous girl I was at thirteen when we first met. He treats me like I've never been sick, and even though that doesn't necessarily align with the way I see myself or feel, it makes me want to play the part. And for a while I do. I play the part so well that I almost trick myself into believing it's the truth.

Although I can't admit it to myself, I'm as seduced by Jon as I am by the idea that a new relationship will help expedite my return to the kingdom of the well. Over the next few weeks, I cannot see him often enough. I join him on tour for a couple of days. We wander around strange cities hand in hand, talking for hours and making shy declarations on park benches. We stay out all night with his friends, bopping from jazz club to jazz club until dawn. I never let on how exhausted I am, I never say no, determined to prove I can hang like everyone else.

But back in New York, when we spend our first night together at my apartment, I am as shaky and uncertain as a lamb. It was one thing to be intimate with Will, who witnessed my body undergo the metamorphosis of illness; it is another thing entirely to be intimate with an outsider, a civilian. As we undress, I feel exposed and insecure. My body reveals a different story to the one I've been presenting: I've lost nearly twenty pounds from the recent bouts of *C. diff,* and my ribs protrude through thin flesh. Bruises and needle marks from IV lines, injections, and blood draws cover my arms. Scars whorl my neck and chest from the multiple central venous catheters I've had over the years. And my port: I still have that, too.

A round plastic butte beneath knotted scar tissue, the port juts up conspicuously above my right breast, hard to the touch. I don't know if I should explain why I still have it, or hope Jon somehow won't notice it in the darkened room. There's so much he doesn't know. If things get more serious between us I'll have to delve into the supremely sexy topics of infertility and chemo-induced menopause, among so many others. The mere prospect of these conversations is enough to contemplate celibacy. *Breathe in, breathe out. I don't know how to do this.*

Jon traces a finger from my lips down my neck to the swirl of scars on my chest. Leaning over, he gently touches his lips to my port, then says, "You're the most beautiful woman I've ever met."

The summer feels like falling in love, not only with Jon, but with the promise of a different life. The only problem is, I'm building this new existence on top of the crumbling foundation of my old one. In late August, after not seeing each other for many weeks, Will and I decide to meet. We grab iced coffees from our favorite breakfast spot across the street and head up to the roof of my building. "I have something I need to tell you," I say, as we sit down at a picnic table.

"Me too, but you first," he replies, ever the gentleman.

I came here planning to tell him about Jon. My announcement isn't coming out of nowhere. Earlier in the summer, I'd warned Will that I was thinking about seeing other people, but he wasn't dumb—he knew that by "other people" I meant Jon. I'd mentioned that we had been hanging out, and I remember Will saying, "Let me know when you've tired of your rebound." He seemed confident that it was just a temporary fling. The remark infuriated me, in part because Will didn't seem to mind as much as I'd hoped and in part because so many of his assumptions were right—about my anger at him, about my inability to be on my own. But since then, what started as a rebound had turned into a meaningful relationship and I felt like I owed Will the truth.

I had rehearsed all morning in my head, telling myself that if I could choose the perfect words, if I said everything just right, Will would understand. We would be able to forgive each other and find closure, maybe even lay groundwork for a lasting friendship.

But sitting face-to-face with Will, it's difficult to sustain my denial. My pupils dart from his face to the ground and back again. The truth? Our situation is so much more complicated than what I've made it out to be. I want to believe that we are over, yet we remain deeply entangled: Will is still the person listed under "emergency contact" on all of my medical forms, still the first person I *want* to call when I'm feeling sick or sad or scared. But what I'm about to tell him will make our split total and irrevocable, and for a moment, I don't know if that's what I want.

Trying to work up the nerve to speak, I count down in my head—three, two, one—but when I finally form the words, my sensitive, carefully rehearsed explanations evaporate. "You should know that I'm in a relationship and it's serious," I say.

Will's blue eyes splinter. As I watch the shock unfurl across his face, I feel a sense of horror at myself. Denial allows you to operate within a vacuum, without having to consider the implications of your actions on your own life or on others. The hurt on his face nauseates me. But a shameful part of me also feels gratified. On some twisted, subconscious level, I think I've been wanting Will to experience a sliver of the pain I felt when he moved out. I want to prove that I am not the needy, powerless sick girl I feel like whenever I'm in his presence. I want him to know that there are others who find me desirable. But even more than that, I want his face in all its pain to validate what I've been longing for: proof that he still cares.

Will is silent for a long time. As he regains his composure, his eyes harden. When he finally speaks, he lets me know that after everything he's sacrificed, I am a traitor and a coward for giving up on us so soon. No one will ever love or take care of me the way he did, he says. Anyway he isn't buying this new relationship of mine. He warns that once I finally come to my senses, I'll regret my actions. "You know what's funny?" Will says. "I came here today to tell you that I'm ready to move back in—to give our relationship another chance. But you've made that impossible."

"How dare you," I hiss. "You don't get to leave me when I'm sick only to swoop back into my life just as I'm finally doing okay."

"Cool, then I guess that's that. Good luck to you and to my replacement," Will replies, stretching his arms over his head and yawning in an exaggerated way.

We had both made fatal assumptions: I never believed he would move out when I issued an ultimatum; Will never thought that once he had, I'd move on. But there is no undoing what's already happened. Neither of us can see past the other's betrayals. Both of us are hurting but feigning indifference. We're each too proud to ask for or grant forgiveness.

I stay on the roof for a long time after Will leaves. I am disoriented and unsure of everything: the sky, the pigeons, the blare of sirens in the distance. Most of all, myself. And yet, about this I feel certain: As much as I can't imagine a life without Will, I can't imagine a way forward with him either. We both need to free ourselves from codependence—from our old roles as caregiver and patient—but I don't see us achieving that together, at least not anytime soon. In order for us to forge new identities, we have to go our separate ways.

Even so, I'm stunned by how quickly we've transitioned from being a pair, utterly enmeshed and in love, to two strangers siloed in private grief and anger. As we set about disassembling what's left of us, it feels less like the final stages of a breakup than the beginning of a gutting, protracted divorce. Will returns his copy of the apartment keys. We close our joint bank account and cancel our family cellphone plan. We sort out shared belongings and although we never ask them to, our respective friends and families sort themselves as well.

As for Oscar, we agree on a joint custody arrangement whereby I take care of him during the week and Will has him on weekends. The first several times we do this, Will rings the doorbell and comes inside to retrieve Oscar. Then one day, he notices a pair of men's size thirteen Air Jordans in the front closet. After that we meet in neutral territory for drop-offs. Soon, Will starts skipping his weekends altogether. It's too hard, he eventually confesses. He, too, needs to start moving on.

Moving on. It's a phrase I obsess over: what it means, what it doesn't, how to do it for real. It seemed so easy at first, too easy, and it's starting to dawn on me that moving on is a myth—a lie you sell yourself on when your life has become unendurable. It's the delusion that you can build a barricade between yourself and your past—that you can ignore your pain, that you can bury your great love with a new relationship, that you are among the lucky few who get to skip over the hard work of grieving and healing and rebuilding—and that all this, when it catches up to you, won't come for blood.

As summer turns to autumn, I begin to feel impatient about my port, the last vestige of cancer that I can touch and see in my body. My medical team insists that it stay in until they are sure I will no longer need it. But I want to be able to wear whatever I please without worrying about people staring at the weird disc bulging below my collarbone; I want to be rid of what feels like the last remaining barrier between me and normalcy. At my next checkup at Sloan Kettering, I bring up the topic of its removal again. After all, it's been five months since my last day of chemo. I've had lots of minor scares since then—resulting in three colonoscopies and three endoscopies, the occasional X-ray, and a bone marrow biopsy following an alarming, mysterious dip in my blood counts—but for the most part, my health has been relatively stable. After discussing it among themselves, my medical team agrees and schedules a date for me to have it removed the following week. It is a vote of confidence in my ability not only to *be* healthy but to *stay* healthy. I am elated.

On a Friday in late October, Jon and I head to Sloan Kettering for the procedure. After seeing firsthand how illness can erode a relationship, I've tried to distance him from all things medical. I even hide my pillbox whenever he's staying at my place and wait until he isn't around to take my medications. I do not expect or ask for much of anything—I ruined my last relationship by needing too much—but hospital rules dictate that someone must be there to bring me home from surgery.

"Here are the face masks and gloves," I explain to Jon in the waiting room. "Yes, you need to wear them, too—it's to protect the other patients who have compromised immune systems." It's strange to fill him in on customs that are second nature to me. I keep glancing over at him, analyzing his body language, looking for signs that the whole cancer thing freaks him out, but Jon seems unfazed.

A nurse comes over and asks me some preliminary questions before taking me to the operating room. Among the usuals— current medications? new symptoms? pain?—she throws a couple of curveballs: "I see in the notes that you were last hospitalized for *C. diff* and possible GVHD of the intestines," she says. "Are you continuing to experience frequent nausea? How many bowel movements are you having a day? What about your stool consistency? Still loose?"

I'm so mortified at this point that I'm harboring murderous impulses—but if Jon is repulsed, he doesn't show it. When it's time for me to be wheeled away, he kisses me through my mask and tells me he'll be there when I wake up.

On the operating table, I lie in a backless hospital gown under a blaze of fluorescent lights. "Congratulations!" the surgeon says to me as he enters. "I hear you are being deported today." He is referring to the removal of my port, of course—the gateway for the dozens of rounds of chemotherapy, antibiotics, stem cells, immunoglobulin, and blood transfusions that have entered my body since diagnosis. It's a line he's clearly delivered dozens of times, a routine intended to make patients smile. As problematic as the pun is, this moment does feel like an official eviction of sorts, a final procedure that will firmly deposit me back in the kingdom of the well.

An anesthesia mask is strapped over my face and I am told to count down from ten. "See you on the other side," the surgeon says before I drift into a deep, chemical sleep.

I wake up in the recovery room forty-five minutes later. My nerve endings bristle and tingle as I rouse from the twilight. Lids fluttering open, pupils rolling around the room like marbles, I can't quite figure out where I am or why Jon, and not Will, is sitting in the chair next to my hospital bed. Then I see the bandage on my chest and remember what has happened. Instead of relief, I feel bereft at the loss of my port—at the thought that now my visits to Sloan Kettering will be fewer and farther between, that I won't get to see my favorite nurses and doctors as often. The sadness is the start of something too complex and discomfiting for me to parse quite yet. So I chalk it up to the aftereffects of the anesthesia.

Later that night, Jon suggests we go out to celebrate. I still feel off, but I make an effort to rally. We get dressed up and go to a gala at the Apollo Theater. Jon, who's become somewhat of a celebrity among the Harlem cultural elite, keeps getting pulled away from our table by people who want to chat or to snap a selfie with him. I sit alone for much of the night downing goblets of chardonnay. At one point, the bandage on my chest detaches, slithering down past my navel and the hem of my dress before plopping onto the floor. I discreetly kick it under the skirt of the tablecloth, looking around to see if anyone noticed. My exposed stitches, tender and raw, rub against the fabric of my dress. I try to ignore the pain as I watch couples glide around a black-and-white-checkered dance floor, but it doesn't work. The sight of these gowned women and tuxedoed men glittering under a canopy of soft white string lights makes the edges of the room where I sit seem gloomier, lonelier somehow. When I raise my hand to my face, I'm startled to discover my skin is slick. Tears mixed with mascara run down my cheeks in big, inky drops.

"What's wrong?" Jon says in alarm when he returns. It's a question he'll ask me repeatedly in the coming months, shocked to discover that the happy, confident, game-for-anything woman he fell in love with is an aspirational act.

What I say in response: "I'm fine."

What I want to say but don't know how to articulate: My port has been removed but it's not gone. Its absence is a new kind of presence, a realization of all the other imprints of illness with which I have yet to contend. The ravages of treatment on my brain, my body, my spirit. The toll of burying dead friend after dead friend and the grief that's been accumulating, unattended, inside of me. The heartbreak of losing Will and my fear that I've made a mistake in not taking him back. The terror and utter confusion I feel about what to do next.

After three and a half years, I am officially done with cancer—more than four years, if you start with the itch. I thought I'd feel victorious when I reached this moment—I thought I'd want to celebrate. But instead, it feels like the beginning of a new kind of reckoning. I've spent the past fifteen hundred days working tirelessly toward a single goal—survival. And now that I've survived, I'm realizing I don't know how to live.

The hero's journey is one of the oldest narratives in literature. Survivors, like heroes, have faced mortal danger and undergone impossible trials. Against all odds, they persevere, becoming better, braver for their battle scars. Once victory has been secured, they return to the ordinary world transformed, with accrued wisdom and a renewed appreciation for life. For the past few years, I've been bombarded with this narrative, observing it in movies and books, fundraising campaigns and get-well cards. It's hard not to traffic in such clichés when they've become so culturally embedded. It can be even harder not to internalize them and to feel as if you have to live up to them.

Over the fall, I make attempts to inhabit that narrative, to return to living as triumphantly as I can. I drag myself to the gym in the basement of my building a couple of times a week—a feat, even for my pre-illness self. I buy a juicer and for a short while force myself to drink gag-inducing kale concoctions. I go to my neighborhood coffee shop each morning and try to write something new. I have moments of laughter and lightness when I go out dancing with friends, but they are brief—gone as quickly as they appear.

But I'm supposed to be better, I repeat endlessly to myself. After all, on paper, I am no longer considered sick. The torrent of doctors' appointments, blood tests, and phone calls from concerned friends and family has slowed to a trickle. Any day now, I will be deemed well enough to be kicked off disability. If I manage to stay cancer-free for a few more years, I might even join the ranks of cancer survivors who are considered "cured." And yet, I've never felt farther from being the healthy, happy young woman I hoped to be on the other side of all this.

Every morning, I still down a fistful of pills. Immunosuppressants prevent my body from rejecting my brother's marrow. Twice-daily doses of antivirals and antibacterials protect my fragile immune system. Ritalin combats the chronic fatigue and fogginess that haven't lifted since the transplant. Levothyroxine does the job of my chemo-ravaged thyroid. And hormone replacements cover for my withered ovaries.

Worse are the psychological imprints of illness, largely invisible to others and devoid of easy fixes. Depression descends like a demon, holding me captive for days, sometimes weeks at a time. Anxiety surges as I wait to hear the results of a routine blood test.

Panic overtakes me each time I see a missed call from the doctor's office or discover a mystery bruise on the back of my calf. Grief continues to haunt me, Melissa's Nile-green eyes floating through my dreams, night after night, as I sleep.

The harder I try to find my place among the well, and to live up to my expectations of the survivor's journey, the more I experience a dissonance between what should be and what is.

Even acknowledging this schism feels impossible: I've already put my parents through so much, and I don't want to worry them with the challenges I am facing now. My medical team is focused on cancer, not its aftermath. Painfully aware that the struggles of recovery are a privilege many don't get to experience, I'm afraid of sounding ungrateful—or worse yet, insensitive to those dealing with far scarier unknowns.

But the contradictions leave me mired in unanswerable questions: Will my cancer return? What kind of job can I hold when I need to nap four hours in the middle of the day, or when my misfiring immune system still sends me to the emergency room on a regular basis? My editor is ramping up pressure for me to resume the column; readers want to know how I am doing, she prods, to hear about life after cancer. But whenever I sit down to write, I can only churn out lies. I want to give readers the kind of narrative resolution both they and I have hoped for all these years—to be able to say that Will and I are still together, that our long-postponed wedding is finally under way; that I'm now training for a marathon, reporting investigative features from far-flung locales, and having a baby. But, of course, that would be fiction.

Because I can't reconcile what I imagined remission to look like with the facts of my reality, I put the column on permanent hiatus. I stay financially afloat by drumming up some speaking engagements and taking a part-time job at a real estate investment company that I'm able to do remotely from bed, but the work isn't sustainable or fulfilling. I barely ever see friends, and when I do, I brace myself for the dreaded three questions: How is my health? What happened to Will and me? What will I do next? Eventually, I stop going out altogether.

Meanwhile, Jon's career is skyrocketing. He has always been the hardest-working person I know and I'm so proud of his success, but being in a relationship with a touring musician who spends more time on the road than at home is rough. I don't feel safe in my own body yet without a constant companion or caregiver by my side and whenever I'm alone, I fall apart. At the same time, whenever Jon is around, I keep him at arm's length. These mixed messages are confusing, and soon he begins asking for more. He wants to know where our relationship is going. He wants to know my thoughts on marriage and children. He wants me to open up. But the gap between us only widens the more he asks.

When Jon goes out of town for a gig, I crumple into bed, exhausted from the effort of pretending I'm okay. I pull the comforter over my head and curl into my usual position: fetal. I let myself cry—ugly, shuddering sobs. I stay in bed like this for days with the drapes closed, ignoring emails and phone calls, leaving my apartment only when the dog whines. Each night, I fall asleep telling myself that tomorrow will be the day when I finally get it together. Each morning, I wake up feeling so sad and lost that I can barely breathe. In my lowest moments, I fantasize about getting sick again. I miss the sense of purpose and clarity I felt while in treatment—the way staring your mortality straight in the eye simplifies things and reroutes your focus to what really matters. I miss the hospital's ecosystem. Like me, everyone there was broken, but out here, among the living, I feel like an impostor, overwhelmed and unable to function.

On an early morning that winter, I am out walking Oscar, wearing the gaunt, zombie look of someone who splits her time between Earth and some other, darker place. As I make my way up

Avenue A, I bump into a man I vaguely recognize from the neighbor-hood coffee shop where freelancers hang out—he's a novelist, I think. He's dressed snappily in a tweed overcoat with leather elbow patches and a briefcase. I'm dressed in my pajamas and smoking a loosie I bought at the corner bodega for fifty cents.

"Wake up, princess," he says, looking me up and down. "Death is the last resort."

I feel so ashamed standing there, under his fixed gaze and the glare of the white winter sun. I've spent the better half of my twen-ties fighting to survive only to become someone so defeated as to elicit a sidewalk intervention from a concerned stranger. During my time in treatment, I'd had one simple conviction: *If I survive, it has to be for something. I don't just want a life—I want a good life, an adventurous life, a meaningful one. Otherwise, what's the point?* And yet, the place I've arrived at is the opposite. Now that I've been afforded the possibility of a good life, I'm not living it—worse, I'm squandering it. Guilt compounds my shame: I know how lucky I am to be alive, when so many I love are not. Out of the ten young cancer comrades I befriended during treatment, only three of us are still here.

As I walk home, it becomes clear: I cannot continue on like this. Something—or maybe everything—must change.

26

RITES OF PASSAGE

THERE IS AN impulse to trace a monumental decision—like embarking on a long journey—back to a single epiphany, a flare of inspiration. A plan of action that arrives fully formed when you find yourself lying on the floor, praying for something, anything, to change.

I do not have one such moment.

My decision to leave home and to go on the road comes to me in stages, but it begins with a trip I take for someone else.

On the one-year anniversary of Melissa's death and the end of my chemo, I stand in the security line at John F. Kennedy International Airport, hoping that the TSA agents won't rifle through my suitcase. With a name like Suleika Jaouad, it's not uncommon for me to get flagged at border crossings and airport security, but for once I actually have something to hide. In my suitcase I've stuffed a vial of gray-white powder inside a pair of socks. This isn't your typical contraband: I'm smuggling some of Melissa's ashes onto a fifteen-hour flight to India.

After Melissa died, a grant was established in her name to send young adults with cancer on a trip abroad. I didn't have to think twice about accepting the first grant—or, when Melissa's parents asked, bringing a piece of her with me to India. The place meant so much to her when she visited, and it was where we had hoped to travel together someday. My decision to go now is a way of commemorating Melissa and a trip that never came to pass. It's also a first exercise in confronting my ghosts.

It wasn't easy to convince my medical team to let me travel to India, given my weak immune system. "The risk of serious infection is too high," my doctor said when I first raised the idea. But he eventually came around and began weaning me from immuno-suppressants so that my body could ward off germs. I had to get a round of vaccinations, undergo a battery of blood tests, and receive sign-offs from everyone on my medical team confirming I was well enough to go.

As I board Air India, I strap a mask across my mouth and sterilize my seat, meal tray, and armrests with antiseptic wipes. But despite such precautions, I fall ill with a virus within a few days of arriving in Delhi. I'm weak and feverish for much of the two weeks I'm there, and end up having to go to a local hospital to make sure it's nothing serious. I'm beginning to understand that no matter how much time passes, my body may never fully recover to what it once was—that I can't keep waiting until I'm "well enough" to start living again. It's a bitter concession but a necessary one. While it might not be possible to move on from illness, I have to start trying to move forward with it.

As terrible as I feel, each day I drag myself out of bed and head outside to explore. I put the vial of Melissa's ashes in my coat pocket and carry it with me everywhere I go, feeling her presence with each step. Together, we explore the dusty streets of Delhi: the pungent spice markets, contemporary art galleries, and sprawling gardens strewn with ruins. We ride rickshaws through a chaotic tangle of buses, bicycles, and the occasional elephant. As we wander, I take on Melissa's painterly gaze, and I relish the vibrancy of the colors—the gem-toned saris, the flower stands filled with marigolds, and the Technicolor pigments that dancing revelers throw into the air by the handful during the Hindu festival of Holi. As part of the grant, I spend each afternoon volunteering at Mother Teresa's Home for the Dying, a hospice for the destitute, where I hang wet laundry on lines of chicken wire and hand out meal trays to the bedridden.

I save the Taj Mahal for last. I've carried Melissa with me for two weeks, and it's time to say goodbye. I arrive one morning before the sun rises: Only a dozen tourists stand in line, waiting for the gates to open. The streets are dark and deserted except for a stray dog sleeping in the middle of the road, her puppies coiled around her for warmth. I tell the tour guide that I have a vial of ashes to scatter once we get inside. The guide informs me that this is against the rules and security is very strict, it will never be allowed. I tell him Melissa's story and how much she wanted to return here. By the time I'm done, the tour guide not only agrees, he offers to smuggle the vial in himself.

The Taj appears like a floating poem in the dawn, a moon-white dream of marble pillars and minarets. It's a place that spoke to Melissa as she faced the end of her life, and after studying its history I understand why. It was commissioned by the Mughal emperor Shah Jahan as a memorial for his wife, who had died giving birth to their fourteenth child in 1631. The emperor was so grief-stricken, the story goes, that his hair turned gray overnight. He vowed to immortalize their love with a monument more beautiful than any the world had ever seen. It took decades to build, but once it was completed, the emperor was able to find solace. As I wander through the ornamental gardens, I think of how the Taj embodies both love and grief. So did my friendship with Melissa. In life, I'm realizing, you don't get one without the other.

Ascending the steps, I drink in the calligraphy and semiprecious stones—coral, jade, onyx—inlaid in marble. I circle around to the back terrace that overlooks the Yamuna, a sacred river flanked by the crackling fires of crematoriums where Hindus come to say last rites for their dead. Gazing onto the river, I think of Melissa's final Instagram post. It was a picture of her taken in India, captioned with the words: *gate gate paragate parasangate bodhi svaha*. Gone, gone, gone beyond, gone altogether beyond, O what an awakening, all hail. I scan the terrace for security officers, and when the coast is clear, I step over the rope cordon and walk to the edge. I open my palm toward the river. For a second, the vial catches the light. Then it tumbles toward the water and is gone.

Taking Melissa's ashes to the place she loved most doesn't lessen the pain of losing her, but it has shown me a way that I might begin to engage with my grief. It has introduced me to the role of ritual in mourning—the ceremonies that allow us to shoulder complicated feelings and confront loss; that make room for the seemingly paradoxical act of acknowledging the past as a path toward the future. It gets me thinking about the other ways we mark the crossing of thresholds: birthdays and weddings and baby showers, baptisms and bar mitzvahs and quinceañeras. These rites of passage allow us to migrate from one phase of our lives to another; they keep us from getting lost in transit. They show us a way to honor the space between no longer and not yet. But I have no predetermined rituals. They are mine to create.

From a distance of several continents, I am able to see my life with clearer eyes. For too long, I've been like a bee trapped inside a window, smashing my forehead against the glass with mounting desperation in a futile attempt to get out. These last two weeks have provided a temporary respite, but I worry that once I'm back home in New York, I'll return to that sad, stuck state. I feel I have to do something drastic to ensure I won't.

On the long flight home, I daydream about embarking on a solo pilgrimage, though what form it might take, I don't know. I want to be in motion—to figure out a way to unmoor myself, to thrust myself into the greater expanses of the world. Not because I have a particular hankering to explore, but precisely because I've grown afraid of the world and my ability to navigate it alone. I want to expect nothing. To ask for nothing. To depend on no one. To find out what lies on the other side of the in-between place. To start living again.

I don't yet have the vision, strength, or resources to cast off on an epic journey, so I begin my quest with a series of short, preliminary outings. A few weeks after I return home, I board a train to Vermont, where my family owns a little log cabin near the Green Mountains. I had always been too unwell to come here alone. Now, though, learning how to be on my own feels like a necessary first step to whatever is next. I need to trust that I can be independent. I need to become my own caregiver. It took me a while to say I was a cancer patient. Then, for a long time, I was only that. It's time for me to figure out who I am now.

Buried deep in the woods, the cabin has no cellphone reception, and the nearest town is a fifteen-mile trek down a desolate highway, past flaxen cornfields, dense stands of trees, and the occasional farm. With the exception of a neighbor, Jane, who is retired and lives with her husband a mile down the dirt road, I don't know anyone. Since I still lack a driver's license, Jane offers to pick me up from the train station. She takes me to the supermarket so I can load up on provisions and then drops me at the cabin, where I stay until I run out of food. "Honey, you sure you'll be okay out here all by yourself?" she asks, concern splayed across her face. Other than Oscar, it's just me, the deer that graze beneath the apple tree, and the sloping spines of the mountains in the distance.

"I enjoy the solitude," I reply, with an air of false confidence. The truth is, I'm terrified of what will happen when I'm alone with my thoughts.

Jane drives away, and I unpack my things, then settle into an armchair near the stone fireplace and try to read. But I'm anxious and can't seem to focus. The quiet and isolation have a magnifying effect, and I see more clearly than ever just how fearful and fragile I've become. Each hoot and howl echoing from the woods makes me jump, and I wake in the middle of the night to triple-check that the front door is locked or that there isn't a serial killer lurking behind the woodpile on the porch. In my life B.C.—before cancer—I was obstinately independent and prided myself on my moxie, whether it was studying abroad in Egypt, reporting from the Gaza border, or hitchhiking across the Jordanian desert. My escapades often crossed over into recklessness. But living with a life-threatening illness for so long has changed my relationship to fear. It has trained me to be on high alert for the countless potential dangers lurking in my body and beyond.

I am jittery and uncomfortable virtually every minute of this first trip to Vermont, but I force myself to live by a rule: I am not allowed to leave out of fear. In moments when all I want is to flee back to the city, I resolve to stay for an extra night, then two, then three. I decide to trust that what feels unknown and frightening will soon feel familiar and safe. I tell myself that, with enough time, I'll grow tired of triple-checking the lock or losing sleep over imaginary predators. Maybe I will even start to make good on my lie to Jane—I might start to enjoy being alone. By the time I head back to the city on day four, I'm not quite there, but getting closer.

Over the next couple of months, I return to Vermont as often as possible. With each trip I take to the cabin alone, I begin to feel

a little more self-possessed, a little more brave, a little more curious about what lies outside the window. I walk longer and longer
distances with Oscar, who sprints ahead, leading me down winding country roads, past ramshackle barns, bubbling streams, and
riverbanks padded with emerald-colored moss. I learn to build a
fire and venture deep into the woods to gather kindling. One day,
a black bear lumbers onto the property and Oscar leaps up from
the porch, roaring at it with the ferocity of a lion. The bear is so
startled that it stumbles and trips, then breaks into a sprint and
disappears behind the tree line. "The courage of children and
beasts is a function of innocence," Annie Dillard once wrote. "We
let our bodies go the way of *our* fears."

Entire days pass when I don't see anyone. I call Jon from time to
time, but he's busy, back on tour. He also seems to understand—
without me even explaining it—that I'm working through something big and daunting, and that what I need most is time alone.
My solitude is interrupted only by sporadic visits from a young
man named Brian who comes by to plow the long driveway and, as
the weather gets warmer, to help out with the garden. One day, we
get to chatting and when he finds out that I don't know how to
drive, he offers to teach me. In exchange for our lessons, I lend him
a sympathetic ear, listening as he tells me about the difficulties of
coming out in rural Vermont, and his various adventures on a gay
networking app called GROWLr. We brainstorm ideas for his dating profile. "Cubbish, bearded, two hundred and thirty pounds,
average looks. Big heart, hopeless romantic. Favorite flower: al-
lium," Brian says.

I suggest: "Well-endowed Gemini."

He erupts with laughter. "Actually, I'm a Leo."

Brian is the closest thing I have to a friend around here, and I
look forward to his company, if not the part where I actually have
to get behind the wheel.

Learning to drive was a momentous high school milestone for most of my friends, who, on the morning of their sixteenth birthdays, rushed to the Department of Motor Vehicles to get their permits. To them, and to most other American teenagers, driving was the ultimate coming-of-age ritual. It meant making out in the backseat late at night, giving your friends lifts to the mall, and tailgating at concerts. It meant independence. But to me, driving just sounded like a terrifying and overwhelming responsibility. A couple of disastrous trial runs in my parents' minivan confirmed what I'd already suspected: It was best for pedestrians, cyclists, and drivers everywhere if I didn't learn at all. It was no coincidence that I'd chosen to go to college in a small town where a car wasn't necessary and then, after graduation, to live in big cities where the go-to transportation was the subway.

Being in Vermont without a driver's license, however, is more than inconvenient. I dislike having to ask for rides, which only reminds me of my dependence. When I run out of milk for coffee, I want to be able to drive myself the twenty miles to the farmers market. It isn't so much that I've stopped being afraid but that my fear is slowly being supplanted by a yearning for freedom.

All summer, Brian gives me lessons, and I learn to navigate the back roads and practice parallel parking between pine trees. As I get more comfortable behind the wheel, a hazy idea begins to crystallize into a grand plan. My time in India has given me a glimpse into how travel can hurtle you out of old ways of being and create conditions for new ones to emerge. It's becoming clearer and clearer to me that I need to leave the familiar, but I don't want to do it entirely alone—I want to seek out others who can offer perspective into my predicament, who can help guide my passage. By the time I finally pass my driver's test, the next step is obvious: I am going to go on a road trip and visit those who sustained me when I was sick.

.   .   .

It's nearly midnight, the logs in the fireplace reduced to ash, but I rekindle the embers and make a pot of coffee. Sitting on the cabin floor, I open a large hand-carved wooden box I bought many years ago from an antique store. In it are birthday cards from my grandmother, photographs, ticket stubs, and macabre medical mementos, like old hospital bracelets and my port. The box also contains hundreds of letters. There are beat-up envelopes sent from faraway lands, love notes etched onto bar napkins, thick stationery stock inscribed with invitations, and dozens of faded printouts of emails. Some of these dispatches were sent to me by people I know well, like Will's father. He wrote me more than two hundred postcards—one every day of that first long summer after my diagnosis and one every day following my transplant until I was in the clear. But most of them were sent to me by people I'd never met.

They say that in difficult times you find out who your friends are, but mostly I found out whom I wanted to befriend. Some people I thought I could count on disappeared, while others I barely knew did more than I ever expected. I was floored by the thoughtfulness of these strangers—readers of the column, anonymous commenters on the Internet, hospital waiting room acquaintances, and friends of friends I barely knew—who sent me care packages and humorous emails, confessional Facebook messages and long handwritten letters. They were more honest and vulnerable with me than a lot of the people I knew off-line. They shared their own stories about what it's like to have life interrupted, whether by the rip cord of a diagnosis or some other kind of trauma or heartbreak. They taught me that, when life brings you to the floor, there is a choice: You can allow the worst thing that's ever happened to you to hijack your remaining days, or you can claw your way back into motion.

Since finishing treatment, I'd found myself gravitating toward the box. There was one letter in particular that I liked to read. It was a printout of an email from Ned, the twenty-five-year-old who wrote to me when I was living at the Hope Lodge in 2012 about the difficulty of transitioning back to "the real world." The message angered me when I first received it; it arrived around the time I learned that I was going to have to resume chemo after my transplant. *What could possibly be so hard about transitioning back to normality?* I'd thought. *All I want is normality.* But once I'd emerged from the fog of treatment, I saw that Ned was right. As I attempted my own rocky passage, I turned to the letter repeatedly, finding comfort in his words. I knew very few people in real life who understood what it was like to be trapped between two worlds.

There were many others who had written to me, and who could maybe offer insights into what it meant to live again in the aftermath of catastrophe. There was Howard, the retired art historian in Ohio, who'd spent most of his life struggling with a debilitating health condition and had built a vibrant life nonetheless. There was Bret, the young man whom I'd briefly met the first time I'd gone to chemo alone and who was now recuperating and attempting to restart his life back home in Chicago. There was Salsa, the ranch cook who'd offered to pile my supper plate high if I ever found myself in Montana. There was Katherine, the high school teacher in California who was attempting to continue on after her son's suicide. And, of course, there was Lil' GQ, the Texas death row inmate whose careful cursive—those looping *p*'s and *q*'s inked in blue on frayed notebook paper—remained tattooed on my memory: *I know that our situations are different, but the threat of death lurks in both of our shadows.*

As I sift through the box's contents, I make a list of two dozen people whose words and stories have kept knocking around my head. I draft letters to each of them. I explain that I'll be embarking on a road trip and ask if they might be open to meeting. I'm not sure what to expect as I hit Send. In most cases, it's been years since they initially reached out to me and I often wasn't well enough to respond. I have no idea if they will remember me—or if they are still alive. But to my great excitement, within a few days, my in-box fills with a near-unanimous chorus of replies inviting me to visit.

I buy a sheaf of road maps and spread them across the kitchen table. Tracing my finger along the curving purple lines of interstates, blue squiggles of rivers, and green swaths of national parks, my itinerary springs to life. The drive will sweep in a counterclockwise circle around the country, going from the Northeast to the Midwest, through the Rocky Mountain states, down the West Coast, and across the Southwest and South, then finally back up the East Coast. I'll travel roughly fifteen thousand miles, drive through thirty-three states, and visit more than twenty people. Oscar and I will go to a boarding school in Connecticut, an artist's loft in Detroit, a ranch in rural Montana, a fisherman's cottage on the Oregon coast, a teacher's bungalow in the Ojai Valley, and an infamous prison in Livingston, Texas. We will go where the letters take us and see what we find.

Over the next couple of weeks, I return to New York to pack all of my belongings into boxes, put the boxes into storage, and sublet my apartment. I can't afford to buy my own car but my friend Gideon generously offers the use of his old Subaru. Between the extra income from renting out my apartment and the four thousand dollars I've saved up, I should be able to make do. I plan to camp and crash on couches as often as possible, only staying in the occasional motel room. I scour Craigslist for secondhand camping gear and buy a portable propane gas stove, a subzero sleeping bag, a foam bedroll, and a tent. I pack all this, along with a crate of books, a sack of dog food, a first-aid kit, and a camera, into the back of the car. Before leaving, I go in for a last checkup with my oncologist.

My trip will last one hundred days. It's the maximum amount of time my medical team has agreed to until my next follow-up appointment, but I like to think of it as another Hundred-Day

Project, a commitment to daily acts of newness intended to stretch the self. It will be my way of reclaiming a number that, during the countdown to Day 100 after a patient's bone marrow transplant, represents a critical turning point in recovery. The difference, this time, is that the rite of passage is of my own making.

27

REENTRY

IN THE MORNING mayhem of Midtown Manhattan, I finish loading my gear into the car and strap myself into the driver's seat. Oscar sits in the back, emitting anxious, asthmatic pants, his little body trembling so much that I can hear his tags clinking. I try not to take his trepidation personally. Oscar doesn't have a lot of experience in cars—though in fairness, neither do I. *Signal, check mirror, watch for blind spots.* I chant Brian's instructions like a phone number I'm scared of forgetting.

I twist the key in the ignition. As the engine hums to life and I pull out into traffic, I can hear the blood pounding behind my ears. Turning right onto Ninth Avenue, I pass an overflowing trash bin, abandoned bicycles chained to a lamppost, and a heavyset, wild-eyed man in tattered clothing who's standing in the middle of the bike lane. He appears to be waving at me—a sight that strikes me as odd but unremarkable for New York City. As I cruise past, the man's wave intensifies, his arms flapping frantically over his head. He seems to be trying to warn me of something. Before I can give any more thought as to what, car horns begin to scream. And then it hits me: The cars are honking at me. And they are driving straight toward me.

It is minute five of my fifteen-thousand-mile road trip and I'm driving in the wrong direction on a one-way street. I crank the wheel left. I slam a foot onto the accelerator. In a sweeping U-turn, I swerve across the asphalt narrowly avoiding a head-on collision. As I pull over to the side of the road, adrenaline fizzes through my body. *This road trip is a terrible idea,* I think, watching the traffic fly past. *I'm not ready. Too inexperienced. Too fragile to survive out here. The more responsible thing to do is to call the whole thing off.* But even as I tell myself this, I know that I won't—I can't. To stay is to consign myself to refrains of brokenness forever. To leave is to create a new story of self. Really, it isn't much of a choice.

The detritus of my past litters the streets of Manhattan. It's the city where I was born and the city where I nearly died. It's where I fell in love and where, over the last year, I fell apart. As the city recedes out of sight in the rearview mirror, I'm not sorry to see it go.

My destination for the first night is only a hundred miles north, but I won't reach it until dusk. I get turned around and end up on the Garden State Parkway, heading south instead. Still new to the concept of "blind spots," I make several bad lane changes, resulting in more honking and at least one driver giving me an aggressive middle finger. Overwhelmed, I decide to continue south and stop in a small town on the Jersey Shore for an impromptu lunch date with a friend, then pull back onto the highway, this time headed north. I inch through Greater New York City in rush-hour traffic before gradually reaching the fertile green expanses of Connecticut. Driving is not a physical sport per se, but it feels that way. My wrists ache from gripping the wheel. The tendons in my neck throb. The task of sitting upright and focusing on the shifting variables of traffic requires a level of endurance my body still lacks, and it's difficult for me to imagine how I'm possibly going to withstand another ninety-nine days of this.

By the time I approach Litchfield, the last, tepid rays are filtering through the pine trees. I give my cheeks a succession of quick, light slaps to stay awake. When I arrive at the dilapidated farm where I'm staying, it's almost dark. I park beneath an old willow and stagger out into the crisp autumn air, then fish a flashlight, sleeping bag, and dinner provisions from the trunk. I trudge down a footpath that leads to a row of tiny cottages overlooking a meadow. Inside, mine is bare and drafty, one all-purpose room furnished with mismatched armchairs, a cot covered in wool blankets, and a desk. The place belongs to a friend of a friend who is out of town and has offered to let me stay. On the desk, he's left a bottle of wine and a note urging me to make myself at home.

I contemplate pouring myself a glass and cooking a real dinner but I am too beat, and instead I scarf down a peanut butter and jelly sandwich and shimmy into my sleeping bag. Across the room is a sliding glass door that looks onto the darkening meadow. I watch as night knits over everything. My eyes adjust, and I see small details I hadn't noticed before. The faint silhouette of trees swaying in the wind. The stars pricking the night sky one by one. I count them, attempting to hush my unquiet mind, but sleep eludes me. I can't get comfortable on the mattress, which is hard and craggy as bedrock. As I toss and turn, longing for my own bed, I find myself questioning what I am doing here—or, for that matter, why I'm on the road at all. As the hours tick by, the darkness whispers all kinds of worries into my ears, conjuring the horrible things that could go wrong over these next months. A loud bang outside the cottage sends me lurching forward, my heart cantering wildly in my chest, only to discover that it's just the screen door sprung loose in the wind. I lie back down, feeling pathetic—a grown-ass twenty-seven-year-old woman afraid of the dark.

Oscar, meanwhile, has been fast asleep the whole time. He's curled up on an overstuffed armchair, making a soft puff, puff, *pffft* sound as he dozes. I envy his unself-conscious state of being, the total trust with which he moves through the world, seemingly

unaware that there's danger and death in the pot. I whisper his
name and am relieved when I hear him rouse and jump to the floor.
He lopes across the room, his nails clipping against the cold brick,
then nuzzles his nose against my hand. "Get on up," I say, patting
the cot. Oscar isn't allowed to sleep in bed, and he gazes up at me,
perplexed. I pat the bed again. He crouches low on his stumpy
hindquarters and flings himself into the air, landing on the mattress with an inelegant thud. I work my fingers through the silky
fur behind the ears, down the coarse crest of the neck and over to
the pink mottled skin of his belly. He sighs with pleasure and nes-
tles into my chest. I put my arm around him, and we're buddies
together in the dark of our makeshift camp. His warmth radiates
through the thin cotton of my T-shirt. I close my eyes. When I
open them next, a band of pale orange is rising over the meadow.
Day 2 is here.

At dawn, I leave a thank-you note, lock up, and tromp up the hill
to the car, haggard and bleary-eyed. An hour and a half later, over
two-lane country roads, I arrive at the first address on my list: an
all-girls boarding school called Miss Porter's. White clapboard
Victorian dormitories jut up from manicured lawns, so pristine
and proper that the setting looks as if it belongs in an Edith Whar-
ton novel. Searching the sidewalk, my eyes anxiously skim past
throngs of girls with heavy backpacks rushing to class, until they
land on a vaguely familiar face.

Seeing Ned in the flesh is jarring. I attempt to match the man
before me with the photograph I received three years earlier of the
bald cancer patient sitting shirtless on the edge of a hospital bed.
Present-day Ned has a full head of thick, brown hair and he wears
glasses, a blue collared shirt, and wrinkled slacks that give him the
mature, bookish air of someone far older than his twenty-nine
years. It's hard for me to believe this person was ever sick. He
crosses the street to greet me, and as he does, whatever closeness I

felt to him quickly dissipates. I realize that, away from the intimate glow of our computer screens, we are just two strangers meeting on a sidewalk for the first time.

Ned and I exchange an awkward hug. "I'm so excited to meet you!" he says with a bashful smile. "And my students are, too!" He teaches tenth-grade English here at Miss Porter's, and when we were making the plans for my visit, he asked if I'd meet with his students and share a bit about my trip. "This way," he says, then leads me across campus to a shingled schoolhouse, Oscar bouncing excitedly along.

The dozen or so girls are seated in a semicircle around a wooden table in a small classroom. They look like thoroughbreds, athletic and lithe, with long, glossy ponytails and fleece jackets. I can feel the heat rising to my cheeks and my chest turning splotchy the way it does whenever the spotlight is on me. As I take in the room, I begin to think that there's no audience more intimidating than an online pen pal and a group of teenage girls.

"Good morning, ladies," Ned calls out. "I'd like you to meet a very special guest."

"Hi—I'm Suleika Jaouad," I say. "And this is my dog, Oscar."

At the sound of his name, Oscar squeaks with excitement and his woolly butt begins wap-wap-wapping against the floor. A chorus of oohs fills the room as the girls jump out of their seats to pet him, and I silently thank Oscar for breaking the ice. Once the excitement has abated and Ned has successfully ordered the girls back into their seats, the attention returns to me. I shift uneasily from one leg to the other as I tell them that I'm on a long road trip around the country—a hundred days to be exact. I just left home yesterday, and they're my first stop.

The classroom seems stuffy and confined, and I long to be outside in the fresh air of the courtyard. I swallow hard, feeling exposed, then continue on with the story of how I was diagnosed with leukemia right after college. "I'm now in remission," I say. "I'm taking this time on the road to recover from what I've been

through and to reflect on where I want to go next. During these months on the road, I'll be visiting some of the people who wrote to me when I was sick. Your teacher is one of them."

Ned then tells the girls that he, too, had a similar experience in his early twenties, and after coming across my column, he'd felt compelled to write me a letter. "I remember being cooped up in a hospital room and feeling so isolated and frustrated by all the momentum I had lost," Ned says, turning to me. "Believe it or not, I spent a lot of time fantasizing about getting out and embarking on an epic road trip of my own. But you're actually doing it. And now you're here. Kinda surreal."

The girls gawk at us. They appear stunned, but also softened. It's as if Ned seems less teacher-y, more relatable all of a sudden—a young man not much older than they, who has a life outside of the classroom, who gets sick, who has his heart broken and walks the earth with secrets, just as they do.

In the hour that follows, the girls raise their hands one after another and ask dozens of questions about my road trip and my writing. They nod brightly in encouragement as I speak, which helps settle my nerves. Then they begin to share their own stories. A day student whose parents are from Bangladesh talks about the difficulties of switching between cultures at home and in school. Another talks about how her father unexpectedly died and how much she misses him. A competitive athlete with honey-colored freckles later pulls me aside to talk about her own cancer diagnosis a year earlier. "Before, if you had asked me who I was, I would have identified as an athlete," she says softly. "But now, I'm not so sure, because cancer does a weird thing to you. It takes who you are and what you think you know and throws that all in the trash."

When the bell rings, several linger to chat. "Take me with you," one says. "I want to come, too!" says another. I feel profoundly grateful to Ned and his students. They've looked at me in my shy, shaky nervousness and listened as I confessed to my lack of clarity about what lies ahead. And yet, they seem to believe in what I've set out to do and to see in my road trip something exciting and worthwhile. I don't share their confidence, but they've given me a much-needed boost. Their openness has shown me what can happen when we quit all the bullshit posturing and admit to uncertainty.

After class, Ned and I drop Oscar off at his apartment and walk to the school's cafeteria. We pass a wall of oil paintings, presumably former headmistresses, all austere white women who look as if they stepped straight off the *Mayflower* and into the portraits. The elite boarding schools of New England are governed by rules and traditions that someone like me, who attended public school my entire childhood, can't quite grasp. Ned, on the other hand, was born into this kind of environment. As we eat, he tells me about how he was raised on the campus of the Massachusetts boarding school where his parents taught—teaching is in his blood. His position at Miss Porter's is his first job since dropping out of college to begin treatment. When I ask how it's going, his face deflates. "It seems to be going okay," he says. "The administrators are happy. But I worry I don't measure up to the old Ned. And that makes me feel like a fraud."

"Is that the hope?" I ask. "To go back to being the old Ned?"

"I mean, it would be ideal, but it's just not realistic," he says. He shakes his head.

I open my mouth to speak, then close it. What can I possibly add? Ned has just summed up what's taken me almost a year to untangle for myself. There is no restitution for people like us, no return to days when our bodies were unscathed, our innocence intact. Recovery isn't a gentle self-care spree that restores you to a pre-illness state. Though the word may suggest otherwise, recovery is not about salvaging the old at all. It's about accepting that you must forsake a familiar self forever, in favor of one that is being newly born. It is an act of brute, terrifying discovery.

After lunch, Ned takes me on a walk through residential streets with picket-fence yards, past cornfields, down to a nearby river. I've known him for only a couple of hours, but I find myself speaking more frankly with him than with anyone else in the last year. As we ramble, I tell him about all of it—Will, Melissa, Jon, and the depression that held me hostage. I even tell him about the smoking and my relapse fantasies. For so long, I've been bound by the *omertà* that seems to envelop survivorship, too ashamed to confide the truth in anyone. It is a relief to know not only that Ned will understand but also that he's experienced many of these challenges himself.

"So, I've been meaning to ask—what made you want to come visit me?" Ned says.

"What you wrote to me about transitioning out of treatment—how hard it was going to be—I get it now," I say. We walk silently for a bit and then I add: "I know you can't go back to the person you were before cancer. But I was hoping that you'd found your way back to normality by now."

Ned's pace slows as he listens. I mention Sontag's kingdoms and ask what it's been like for him to reenter the realm of the well. Ned cocks his head, appearing thrown. "I wish I could tell you I've climbed over that barbed wire and made it back," he says. "But honestly I just don't know if that's possible."

His answer is dizzying, and as we continue on, I realize what I'm feeling is profound disappointment. The notion that reentry is an ongoing and difficult process is usually referenced in the context of veterans of war or the formerly incarcerated, not to survivors of illness. Over the last year, I'd imagined Ned settled back into the kingdom of the well, the worries in his letter long behind him, and that he'd now be in a position to guide me. But he, too, is still finding his way, still struggling to carry the collateral damage of illness, and suddenly I realize: We may always be.

"Did you notice anything strange about the way I walk?" Ned asks, pointing out the slight limp in his step.

His limp was the first thing I'd noticed when we started walking, but it doesn't seem polite to say so, so I say nothing.

Ned tells me that a side effect of his chemo regimen was that it eroded his joints, and he recently had both hips replaced. He suffers from neuropathy and chronic pain, which makes it difficult to run or to play sports. And like so many former patients, he lives with a constant hum of vigilance, ears pricked for bad news, eyes ever on alert for signs that disease has re-infiltrated the plot.

I know all about this, I do the same. Before I left, I spoke with a doctor at Sloan Kettering who explained that I was experiencing post-traumatic stress disorder, a diagnosis I had always believed was reserved for people who had endured unspeakable, violent atrocities. Some traumas, I learned, refuse to remain in the past, wreaking havoc in the form of triggers and flashbacks, nightmares and fits of rage, until they've been processed and given their proper place. This helped me understand why the horror of my cancer did not end on my final day of treatment but surged in its aftermath: The haunting feeling that something terrible could happen again at any moment. The nightmares that tore me from sleep. The panic attacks that left me gulping for air on scraped knees. The resistance I felt to forging real intimacy. The private shame that I carried and the guilt that I bore at how all of this affected those around me. The nagging voice in my head that whispered: *Don't get too comfortable because one day I'm coming back.*

Recognition of my post-traumatic stress was a revelation, but so was the possibility of what psychologists describe as "post-traumatic growth." My illness has humbled and humiliated and schooled me, offering knowledge that might otherwise have taken decades for my pre-diagnosis, self-absorbed twenty-two-year-old self to accrue. But that old Hemingway saw—"the world breaks every one and afterward many are strong at the broken places"—is only true if you live the possibilities of your newly acquired knowledge. Neither Ned nor I have quite figured out how to do this, but as we finish our walk and part ways for the afternoon, I feel comforted to know I'm not the only one.

·　·　·

Later that evening, I slide behind the wheel, then pick Ned up for dinner. The car lurches down the highway, the sky turning a darker and darker shade of charcoal. I've never driven on a highway at night before and am reassured to have someone other than Oscar as a co-pilot. Ned directs me to the restaurant, giving driving advice as I change lanes. I'm feeling confident by the time we arrive, and I pull into a parking space, then hop out and start walking toward the restaurant. But Ned remains frozen by the curb. "I feel the need to point out that your car is parked diagonally across two spots," he shouts after me. He's trying hard not to laugh. "Since we're in front of a liquor store, it might be prudent to repark it before someone calls the cops on what appears to be a very sloshed driver."

Once the car has been properly reparked, we head toward the neon red SEOUL B.B.Q. & SUSHI sign. As we wait for the waiter to bring our appetizers, Ned reaches into his backpack and pulls out a manila envelope. He slides it across the table. When I open it, I find a stack of poems, each one annotated in pencil. "One thing I've learned in the midst of all this," he says, "is that I derive sustenance from poetry. I see my experience embedded in what I read and that becomes the language I use to capture it. I've compiled a few of my favorites. They might speak to where you're at—where we're both at right now."

Ned closes his eyes and begins to recite a few lines of a Stanley Kunitz poem called "The Layers."

> *I have walked through many lives,*
> *some of them my own,*
> *and I am not who I was,*
> *though some principle of being*
> *abides, from which I struggle*
> *not to stray.*

Like Ned, reading and writing have been central to me since childhood. After my diagnosis, putting pen to paper was what allowed me to hold on to a sense of self even as I deteriorated—even when I no longer recognized myself in the mirror. It gave me the illusion of control when I'd had to cede so much of it to caregivers. Trying to render the experience in words made me a better listener and observer of not only others, but also the subtle shifts in my own body. It taught me to speak up and advocate for myself. (My medical team joked that every time they made a mistake, I wrote it up in *The New York Times*.) Reporting on my experience granted me a way to transmute suffering into language. It also created a community—delivering me here to see Ned.

I don't think it's an exaggeration to say that writing saved me. No matter what happened, I churned out words, even if they only amounted to a few sentences.

Except this last year.

After I return to my motel room, I keep thinking about the poem Ned recited—about the idea of a "principle of being" that threads through the past, present, and future. When talking with Ned, I noticed how he kept subconsciously referring to himself as split into three selves: pre-diagnosis Ned, sick Ned, and recovering Ned. Whenever I talk about my life, I realize I do the same. Maybe the challenge is to locate a thread that strings these selves together. It strikes me as a challenge better worked out on paper.

For the first time in months, I crack open my journal and start to write. I decide to do this daily, to follow the thread where it leads.

Between Ned and the next person on my list lie seven hundred miles of highway. A more experienced driver, or someone with a deeper reservoir of energy to draw from, might be able to do it in a straight twelve-hour shot. It will take me nearly two weeks. On the morning of Day 3, I wake up in Farmington with a suspicious scratch in my throat. I've been looking forward to camping but I appear to be coming down with a cold, and forecasts warn of a storm.

Ominous purple and black clouds bruise the sky as I pull into a campground in Middleborough, Massachusetts. Stepping out, I feel a drop of rain, then another. The prospect of sleeping with a dog in a tent in the rain when I'm already sick sounds miserable. At the campground office, I rent one of the cabins instead. They form a half circle in a wooded area, overshadowed by two dozen RVs parked in long rows across a field of yellowed grass. It's hardly the wilderness experience I cooked up in my fantasies.

I unpack my gear and sit at the picnic table outside. It is the first truly cold day of autumn and I'm dressed in jeans, a sweatshirt, a black puffy jacket, and a wool hat. Oscar is asleep on my lap, warming my thighs as I examine my map. I'm absorbed in charting the next week's course northward when Oscar abruptly leaps down, growling and baring his teeth at a car that has just pulled up to the cabin next door. Two little dogs wearing matching pink bows jump out. Their owners follow, a young couple in their thirties, and soon make their way over to me.

"I'm Kevin and this is Candy," says the man, who has gel-glazed hair and a silver chain around his neck.

"Suleika," I say. "Nice to meet you."

"Su-what?"

"Su-lake-uh," I enunciate.

"The hell kinda name is that?" replies Kevin. A harsh bark of laughter escapes his lips. "Ain't American, are ya?"

It's unclear to me if this is a sincere question, a joke, or a racist dig. I don't know what to say, so I laugh, too, hating myself a little for it.

"You here by yourself?" asks Candy.

I say yes without thinking and instantly regret not telling them I am here with my boyfriend, Buck, who is out bison hunting and will be back any minute with his guns. That thought is quickly followed by another. I don't need a man to feel safe on the road: I just need to be discerning about whom I engage with and how. In this instance, it means politely wishing my new neighbors a nice rest of the day and retreating to my cabin. I watch through the screened window as Candy and Kevin head back to their car and, to my relief, drive away.

Once they are gone, I wander back outside and stack logs in the fire pit. They're damp. The fire only catches after several tries, but once it does, I watch with satisfaction as the flames leap and lick at the cool air. The rain has ceased and I snap off Oscar's leash to let him run loose. I lie on my back in the dewy grass, stretching my arms out and caressing the blades with my fingertips. The scent of wood smoke seeps into my nostrils.

I doze off and when I awake, it's already dark. A crescent moon hangs above and all I can think is that it looks like a milky finger-nail clipping. Once again, I'm too tired to try out my camp stove, so I fix another peanut butter and jelly sandwich and plop down at the picnic table with the envelope of poems Ned gave me. But before I can start reading, the sound of crunching brambles distracts me. Squinting into the woods, I glimpse a large dog and a large man wearing a flannel shirt stretched tight across a bulging belly. He's lugging a huge blue tarp filled with—*what? Maybe just camping supplies,* I think. *Alternately, could be a cadaver.* He hauls his load onto the porch of the cabin to my right, without so much as a hello. As he takes a seat on the steps, cracks open a beer, and begins to work through a twelve-pack with remarkable speed, I feel uneasy. My hope for a quiet night by the fire evaporates. I take the poems and what's left of my sandwich inside.

I'd prefer to stay in until morning but the cabin has no plumb-ing and the outhouse is about seventy yards away. Before bed, I grab a flashlight and toiletries to make a quick trip to the bath-room, but as I open the door, Oscar darts between my legs and disappears into the night. "Oscar," I whisper once, then again more loudly. "Oscar, dammit, come here." I strobe my flashlight along the outskirts of the woods, pacing up and down in the tall grass, as I call his name with mounting frustration.

"Your dog on the loose?" My beer-chugging, tarp-dragging neighbor has materialized behind me, and his voice makes me jump.

"Yeah, but I've got it under control."

"You need help looking?" he says. It's as though he hasn't heard a word I just said.

"I'm good," I repeat more firmly and walk away.

I've been living so long in the constricted world of illness that it's not just the safety of my body I don't trust but that of the larger world, too. It's hard to know what reasonable fear is—what you can and can't trust. As much as I love Oscar, I'm not about to search for him in the woods with an unsettling stranger. I turn and march back to my cabin. As I do, I hear the thump of a nubby tail against the porch. Sure enough, it's Oscar, a grin stretched across his scruffy face. "I should send you back to the shelter," I grumble, scooping him up and bolting the door behind me.

The next morning, my cold has worsened. My entire body aches and my head feels as if it's filled with wet squelching sand. It's hard not to feel discouraged by the thought that the majority of the trip might be just this—anxious nights, intermittent sickness, and exhaustion chasing me across state lines. I drag myself to the picnic table outside, where I tinker with the camp stove until I finally get it working. Blue flames flicker under a pot of bubbling oatmeal, and as I dig into my breakfast, my neighbor and his dog reappear. "Howdy," says the man, tipping the trucker hat he wears smashed over a greasy mess of curls. "I didn't get a chance to introduce myself. I'm Jeff, and this here's Diesel," he says, pointing to the black Labrador by his side. "I wanted to apologize for last night—I'm deaf and I couldn't really hear you. I made sure to put in my hearing aids today. Glad you made out okay with your dog."

I can see him more clearly in the light of day. His nails are ragged and his cheeks covered in week-old stubble, but his eyes are kind. I feel a stab of guilt: In the last few years, I've been on the receiving end of enough assumptions to know better. Once, on a snowy winter day in Manhattan, a man yelled at me on the bus for not offering my seat to an older woman. *Sir, I know I may look young but I'm sick, I'm on my way to chemo,* I wanted to explain, but didn't. Instead, under several pairs of reproachful eyes, I flushed with shame and vacated my seat.

"How long have you been camping?" I ask Jeff, making an effort to be friendly.

"I've been sleeping in a tent for the last few weeks, but the rain's been real bad, so I moved into a cabin last night."

"Wow. A few weeks?" I say, impressed. "I'm also on a long adventure."

"I guess you could call this an adventure . . . I had to sell my house and I'm having trouble finding a place I can afford, so this is home for now. A lot of folks at the campground are in the same boat. Tough times, but you won't find me complaining."

Jeff and I talk for a while longer. He tells me about the beaches in nearby Plymouth, a town on the coast. "It's real pretty over there," he says. "You should check it out." The weather is warmer today, and since I have nothing else planned, I do. As I walk along the pebbled shoreline, I think about Jeff and Diesel, about how they are going to fare in the winter months without a home. I think about Ned and his students. I think about the people and the miles of highway I have yet to encounter. Oscar chases waves along the edge of the water. Great streaks of pink and orange crisscross the ocean as the sun sinks lower and lower on the horizon.

A few days later, once both the weather and my cold have improved, I search for a place to try out my tent, determined to camp for real before leaving Massachusetts. Noodling up the coast, I reach Salisbury, where I find Pines Camping Area. I park in front of the A-frame cabin at the entrance. A permed helmet of white hair bobs up from behind the reception desk. Its owner is hooked up to a portable oxygen tank. A pack of Marlboro Reds rests on the counter. "Can I help you?" she rasps.

When I ask if there are any available tent sites for the night, she hands me a map of the campground. "Take your pick," she says. "You're the only one here."

The pine trees loom tall above me as I maneuver past vacant RVs toward the edge of the grounds. In the waning light, I move quickly to unpack my tent and set it up. I spread a plastic tarp and the tent's skeleton onto the ground and stand back with arms folded, surveying my equipment. How hard can this be?

Wrestling with the metal rods, I get my answer fast. My secondhand tent had not come with an instruction manual. After several failed attempts, I toss out any romantic notions of the woods as a respite from civilization and pull out my phone, resorting to a YouTube tutorial. A hunter dressed in camouflage with my exact tent model—a Big Agnes Fly Creek—drawls instructions from a forest somewhere in America. I watch and rewind and watch again, scrambling to clip the tarp to the poles just so.

Since I left home a week ago, I haven't gotten very far on the map and little has gone smoothly. But with each stressful situation, I'm exercising new muscles. I have to believe that if I keep striving toward the person I'd like to become—one who is self-sufficient and independent, one who camps fearlessly in the woods—eventually I'll get there. Once my tent is finally set up, I crawl inside with an overinflated sense of accomplishment. Headlamp strapped to my forehead, I open my notebook and uncap my pen. *I'm camping!* I write. *In a tent! Alone!*

28

FOR THOSE LEFT BEHIND

ODD THINGS HAPPEN when you're on a road trip alone. The monotony of driving becomes meditative: The mind unwrinkles. As the usual anxieties and concerns vacate, daydreams flit in. Occasionally, a wisp of an idea appears out of nowhere only to recede, a shimmery mirage in a desert. Other times, an avalanche of memories tumbles forth, loosened by an old song on the radio or a déjà vu–inducing landscape. The interplay between geography and memory becomes a conversation. They spark and spur each other. Sometimes they even lead to unplanned visits.

LIVE FREE OR DIE reads a big blue sign as I cross into New Hampshire. I'm curious about the origin of the state motto. When I stop at a gas station, I learn via a quick Internet search that it was coined by General John Stark, a famous Revolutionary War veteran, in 1809. Debilitating rheumatism had forced him to turn down an invitation to the anniversary of the Battle of Bennington, so he'd sent a message by mail: "Live free or die: Death is not the worst of evils." As someone trying to break out of a life that no longer feels free, the first part of the slogan resonates. But death does feel like the worst of evils, especially for those left behind, who may never find closure in their grief.

I'm reminded that Melissa's parents live nearby, only a short detour from my route. It doesn't seem right to drive by without at least reaching out, so I shoot her mom, Cecelia, a text letting her know I'm in the area. *Last-minute breakfast?* she offers. *I know a place off of 93 in Windham. It's nice, quaint, and has outside tables so we can sit with our dogs.*

Perfect! I respond. *I can be there in an hour.*

Back in the car, I watch the lines of the highway stream past in long white ribbons, remembering the last time we saw each other. It was a year and a half ago, on a warm, blustery April night in Brooklyn. We'd gathered for Melissa's wake, which—in true Melissa fashion—she had insisted we call a "party." Before heading over, I met up with Max, the poet from the pediatric ward, at a Mexican restaurant, where we each downed a beer and a tequila shot for some liquid courage. The wake was held a few blocks away at a cavernous venue that typically hosted art openings, music video shoots, and fashion shows. I remember Max holding my hand as we made our way through the crowd to where our cancer crew stood in a huddle. The room was packed, airless, and hot. A chandelier made of glowing lawn ornaments cast a smoky, scarlet hue. Melissa's paintings covered every inch of wall space. Per her instructions, there were handles of whiskey, forties of beer, and bottles of good wine, and as the booze flowed, the laughter grew rowdy. When it came time for everyone to take a seat—to acknowledge why we'd all gathered—a contained sense of panic filled the room. Up until that moment, the wake could have been mistaken for a surprise birthday party, but it was as if we were all beginning to realize that our guest of honor would never arrive.

That night made Melissa's absence real in a way it hadn't felt before. It also made visual the devastation her death wreaked on her family, friends, and community. Max sat next to me, wide-eyed

and looking a little faint. I wondered what it must feel like for him
to be here, given that he and Melissa shared a diagnosis. Though
he was okay for now, Ewing sarcoma is vindictive, often returning
again and again to pillage the body until its last breath. As if reading my thoughts, Max wrapped an arm around my shoulders and
I leaned my head against his. "I'm getting a grotesque sense of
what my own funeral might be like," he whispered.

A program of performances, readings, and toasts began, punctuated by the sound of muffled sobs. Melissa's father, Paul, spoke
first. "As a parent, there's no greater pain than losing a child," he
said in his strong Irish brogue. "But we take great comfort in the
incredible legacy that Melissa left us through her art, and through
all her wonderful friends. In the last three years, I spent an amazing amount of time with Melissa as she battled this dreaded disease. I consider myself the luckiest dad in the world." He went on
to recount what he described as one of the best days of his life: It
was a beautiful summer afternoon and despite being in the middle
of another round of chemo, Melissa was feeling pretty good. She
took him to the museum, then to lunch in Brooklyn and to see her
friend Chuck, a tattoo artist. "You're getting a tattoo today," Paul
recounted Melissa saying. They opted for matching tattoos of the
traditional Irish claddagh: two hands clasping a crowned heart,
symbolizing love, honor, and friendship—three things Melissa had
in abundance. From there, she took him to a bar across the street,
where some of her friends were playing bluegrass. "One of the
guys handed me a guitar and we started rockin' it out," Paul told
the room, grinning. "Afterward, Melissa grabbed me by the arm
and said, 'Dad, you really are cool, aren't you?' And, let me tell
you, twentysomething-year-olds do not say that to their dads."
Then he picked up a guitar, strummed, and sang an old favorite
folk tune called "Dimming of the Day" before closing his remarks
with a line that said it all: "I will miss her forever."

As speaker after speaker rose to share a memory or a favorite
story, my gaze kept straying to Melissa's mom, who stood off to

the side, appearing shell-shocked. She was dressed in a blazer, and in honor of her daughter's favorite pastime, had fastened a gold marijuana leaf brooch onto one lapel. Her expression struck me. Face blank. Jaw locked. Eyes steeled. She never cried until the end, when it came time for her to take the mic. "Melissa was just amazing . . ." she said, her voice cracking as she began weeping inconsolably. "I was supposed to say more, but I just . . . I can't."

We call those who have lost their spouses "widows" and children who have lost their parents "orphans," but there is no word in the English language to describe a parent who loses a child. Your children are supposed to outlive you by many decades, to confront the burden of mortality only by way of your dying. To witness your child's death is a hell too heavy for the fabric of language. Words simply collapse.

Melissa's greatest worry in the final weeks of her life had been what would happen to her parents once she was gone. I didn't know what to say whenever she brought it up. I didn't know what to tell her parents on the night of the memorial. Other than a quick hug and a hurried expression of condolence, I'd kept my distance, afraid of uttering the wrong thing or breaking down in their presence. What could I possibly offer to ease their pain?

Now, as I drive to meet Melissa's mom for breakfast, I still don't know what to say. We've never spent time together without Melissa. Until today, most of our encounters had taken place in hospital waiting rooms and hallways. Bearing right at exit 3, I pass a field of cows, a white steepled church, and a farm stand piled high with russet potatoes. When I pull up to the Windham Junction Country Store and Kitchen, Cecelia is waiting for me in the parking lot, dressed in a denim jacket and black Converse hightops. She looks just like her daughter, but with glasses and streaks of gray in her shoulder-length black hair. My chest tightens at the sight of her.

We order coffee and sit outside. The thicket of trees bordering the café glows. "It's peak foliage weekend," Cecelia says, as we admire the view. She has with her a schnauzer puppy she recently rescued from a shelter—she tells me that after seeing how much Oscar helped me, she decided to adopt one of her own. "They make everything a little better, don't they?" I say as the two dogs begin to play.

"They do," Cecelia tells me. "But I won't lie to you: It's been a miserable year. Paul and I have been thinking about packing up and moving. We need a fresh start. We're thinking California or Arizona, but who knows if it'll happen."

My face brightens at the thought of them retiring somewhere with palm trees where the sun shines all year. "Why not do it?" I ask.

"We haven't been able to clean out the house since Melissa died," she confesses. "It's a mess—I'm talking near-hoarder status—and it's embarrassing. That's why I asked you to meet me here instead. We want to move, but we just have so much stuff and I don't know where to start. What am I supposed to do with her old rocking horse? What about her paintings? Her clothes?"

I can't pretend to have solutions for Cecelia's predicament. The task of determining what to keep or give away is difficult enough to do for one's self, let alone on behalf of a child who has died. It's a task that seems to bore into the very meaning of grief, into the anguished battle between holding on and letting go, between staying moored to the past and allowing pieces of it to drift away. But I am certain Melissa would not want them to live in a mausoleum of her old things. In one of our last conversations, when I'd asked Melissa if she was afraid of dying, she replied: "My biggest fear is that my parents' lives will be ruined forever."

"Melissa would want for you and Paul to find a way to continue on. To be happy," I say.

"I don't know if we'll ever be happy," Cecelia says. "It's unbearable. Every day, every hour, without her here. The worst part is that other parents treat us like we have some kind of curse, a contagious one. Grief makes people uncomfortable, I guess. They want you to be positive, they want you to quit talking about your dead daughter, they want you to stop being sad. But we will never not be sad. So what do we do?"

After breakfast, Cecelia walks me to my car. She asks where I'm headed next. I tell her I'm on my way to Ohio, but that I might stop to see my folks before I leave the Northeast. "Well, I have a little something to give you," she says, and she hands me a small backpack for Oscar filled with treats, toys, and a portable canine water bottle. Then, reaching into her jacket, Cecelia opens her palm to reveal an antique silver key. She explains it was part of Melissa's collection of knickknacks. I'm moved by the gesture, and I feel a lump rise in my throat. I don't want to cry, so I choke it down, fish my car keys out of my pocket, and add hers to the ring. "This way Melissa can ride with me as I drive around the country," I say.

Cecelia's waving silhouette slowly disappears as I roll away from Windham. As soon as she is gone from view, tears swarm my eyes. By the time I cross into Vermont an hour or so later, I'm crying so hard that the asphalt and trees blur together. I notice a small clearing off to the side of the road and pull over, killing the engine. I haven't cried over Melissa since the day I learned she died. And now that I'm crying, I can't seem to stop. I thought I'd made peace with her death—at least, as much as was possible—but in this moment, I feel raw in grief. Time, they say, heals all wounds. But Melissa's absence is a wound that will not—cannot—heal. As I get older, she stays dead.

It is the certainty of never that hurts most. The knowledge that I will never eat star-shaped peanut butter and jelly sandwiches with her in the pediatric ward again. Never dance around her living room, headbanging our wigs to the beat. Never watch her paint a new masterpiece. I understand why people believe in the afterlife, why they soothe themselves with the faith that those who are no longer with us still exist elsewhere, eternally, in a celestial realm free of pain. As for me, all I know is that here on this earth, I cannot find my friend.

Hands trembling, I raise my sweater to my face and wipe it dry. Then I drive. Down Vermont's winding back roads littered with fallen leaves. Past cornfields and across covered bridges. I drive until I reach the log cabin where, over the summer, I conceived of this ridiculous trip. I spend a few days sleeping and walking in the woods and weeping some more. Then I continue.

If time has changed anything since Melissa's death, it is that these days, the act of remembering also admits moments of joy, not just sadness. As the car bounces down the dirt driveway, I imagine Melissa sitting in the passenger's seat, bopping her head to the radio, her green eyes glinting in the autumn sun. I ask her opinion on life's dilemmas—on loss and my love life, on how to carry the past into the future and what in the world can be done about my post-chemo mullet—and in my mind's eye, as she smiles yes or shakes her head no, the answers become a little less murky.

While I was talking with Melissa's mother, an intrusive thought kept forcing its way into my mind: *If our stories had ended differently, Melissa could have been the one visiting my grief-ravaged parents.* It's a thought that floods me with a guilt vast enough to drown in—not just that I am here and Melissa isn't, but also that my reentry into the world has so consumed me that I've neglected to think about my own parents' experience. I imagine my mother in Cecelia's position, sitting on the floor of my childhood bedroom surrounded by piles of my things—my favorite stuffed dog, cardboard boxes crammed with report cards and old artwork, my dusty double bass propped up in a corner, and my hand-knit baby clothes carefully folded and wrapped in tissue paper, destined for grandchildren someday. My parents are, of course, fortunate; they haven't lost a child. But living with that possibility, and caring for me through the process, was its own kind of trauma.

Saratoga is an hour's drive from the New York–Vermont border, and at the last minute I decide to stop by my parents' house for a night. I can't remember the last time I visited and as I pull into their driveway, my mother rushes out to greet me. I wrap my arms around her slender shoulders, inhaling the fragrant scent of her face cream. I want to tell her I love her, how much I've missed her, but my family has always been more comfortable with heated dinner table debates than outpourings of affection. It's more than that, though. Over the last year we've stopped talking as frequently or as openly as we used to. In fact, for a time, we weren't talking at all.

I always assumed our closeness would be a constant, especially given everything we went through together. But after I finished treatment, a strange distance emerged. While my parents were aware that my relationship with Will had been strained, no one knew the full extent of our unhappiness and the news of his moving out came as a terrible shock. Will lived in my parents' house for close to a year leading up to the transplant. He joined us on family holidays and spent countless hours sitting with my parents in hospital waiting rooms. After Will and I settled into a place of our own, he stayed in daily contact with my parents, always making sure to text them with health updates and sending them frequent photos. They thought of Will as family, an honorary son-in-law.

More shocking than even our breakup was when I announced to my parents that I was in a new relationship. They were vocal about their disapproval: It was too soon for me to be dating someone new, they said. Was I sure that what was broken between Will and me couldn't be fixed? It was more than six months before they agreed to have dinner with Jon. Slowly, they stopped mentioning Will so often and they made an effort to be more supportive, but I could sense their lingering concern. Where I saw a chance at a fresh start, my parents saw peril—the possibility that I was setting myself up for more heartbreak with a new man who didn't understand how tenuous my health still was.

And that's what every conversation boiled down to—panic about my health. Whenever I was on the phone with my parents and happened to cough or mention fatigue, their replies were laced with apprehension: "Are you sick? Can you make an appointment to get your blood counts checked? Why don't you come home for a rest?" Their worry had become a tic they couldn't help themselves from expressing. They wanted to protect me, but their anxiety could be overwhelming. It hadn't been a conscious decision, but gradually I'd stopped calling or visiting as much. I let emails and texts go unanswered for days; sometimes I didn't answer at all. I knew this was hurtful, especially to my mom, who was used to being in daily contact, but I didn't know what else to do. To quell my own fears, I needed space from theirs.

I follow my mom into the kitchen, where we make turmeric tea, and then we bring our mugs upstairs to her studio. Classical music floats from an old paint-splattered boom box in the corner. The windowsills are covered in shells, branches, feathers, and animal bones that she collects during her daily walks in the woods with my father. On the walls hang her latest creations: giant black-and-white paintings of what appear to be abandoned birds' nests.

We take a seat at the large drafting table pushed up against one of the windows. It's covered in notebooks, jars of paintbrushes, and dozens of tubes of paint, and as my mom clears a space for our mugs I notice her hands. Years of painting and gardening have left them weathered, her fingers knotted like gingerroot, her palms as rough as tree bark. They are the hands that held me right after my birth. They are the hands I glared at with red-hot resentment when it was time for my nightly chemo injections during the clinical trial. They are the hands that changed my urine-soaked sheets when I grew so ill that I wet the bed. Those hands and I have struggled through a lot.

"*Maman?*" I say. "*Merci.*"

"*Pour quoi?*"

"For always taking such good care of me."

"You don't need to thank me. That's what parents do." She looks hesitant for a moment, then adds, "You know what's weird? In terms of my daily life, I was functioning almost better when you were very sick. We were in emergency mode and I had one focus: taking care of you. I couldn't admit how afraid I was that you might not make it. It's only now that you're better that I'm allowing myself to feel my fear—that I'm listening more to what the whole thing has meant."

It's the first time my mom has shared any of this with me—my first glimpse of what the past four years have been like for her. From the day of my diagnosis, she and my dad were beside me. My suffering has been theirs, my disappointments and heartbreaks and uncertainty theirs, too. I imagine it will be a long time before they are able to shake the worry that it could happen again. I'm not the only person in my family trying to move forward.

"You can't keep going and doing the same things as before when everything in your life has been turned upside down," my mom says. "I haven't yet found a journey like the one you're on to help me refocus."

The next morning, my parents and I have breakfast at a family friend's nearby apple orchard. During the meal, the mood is hopeful, but I can sense an undercurrent of concern—though, this time, it's not about my latest blood counts, but instead my ability to use a turn signal. Back at the house, I pack up the car. I wish I could stay longer, but I need to get back on the road. "My Hundred-Day Project is going to be to call you every day," my mother says, poker-faced, as I climb into the car. She stands next to my father, whose hands are clasped conspicuously behind his back. As I pull out of the driveway, I see him step behind my car and splash a glass of water onto the rear windshield. It's an old Tunisian tradition he's done countless times before: to throw water behind a loved one as they venture out on a long trip, a blessing to ensure their safe return.

29

THE LONG FORAY

EITHER MY GPS is a liar or I am an erratic driver, but I always seem to take nearly twice as long as it predicts to get to where I'm going. "Take a right turn in—*recalculating . . .*" its robotic voice says condescendingly when I miss yet another exit. My next destination, Columbus, Ohio, will entail my longest drive yet. The GPS predicts that, if I follow its barrage of orders exactly as told, I will arrive in nine hours and twenty-one minutes. Unlikely.

These days I'm on no one's clock but my own.

Two weeks earlier, when I first left home, I was so tense that I regularly had to remind myself to breathe. Each minute behind the wheel presented new and overwhelming scenarios: Do I have the right of way? What does a blinking red light mean? Was that an Egyptian hieroglyph on the traffic sign? Lane changes and merging onto the freeway had proven especially stressful—an existential guessing game of will I live or will I not. But with each day, I am feeling more confident, and it has been at least seventy-two hours since another driver has honked at me in anger or bewilderment.

Before I left Saratoga this morning, my father showed me how, if I leaned forward in my seat while glancing into the side mirror, the curvature in the glass would allow me to see cars hiding in the blind spot. Now, as I roll along the interstate, miles fly by with newfound ease. Even Oscar seems more relaxed as he gnaws on a bone in the backseat.

After about three hours, I begin to flag, drowsy from the warm sun streaming through the window. Removing my shoes at a rest stop, I recline the seat as far as it can go and stretch my toes onto the dashboard. My fatigue continues to chase me, but instead of fighting it or chastising myself for my slowness, I close my eyes under the golden arches of a McDonald's. I am trying not just to accept my body's limitations for a change, but to savor the breaks I have to take because of them. These pit stops end up being some of my favorite moments on the road—shifting me out of my swirling mind and into the present, anchoring me in this strange new body, and in new places where I otherwise would never have gone.

A half hour later, I awake, revived. I'm able to log another 150 miles before I decide to break for the day. I find a cheap motel on the outskirts of Buffalo, and as I wait for the receptionist to fetch my room key, I skim through brochures advertising boat trips along Niagara Falls. It's a gray, dreary day. Oscar needs exercise but the only greenery in sight is a small strip of desiccated grass encircling the property. We jog loops around the parking lot to the whooshing soundtrack of tires plowing through puddles on the nearby freeway. Out of nowhere, hail begins pelting down on us. Oscar raises his snout and growls at the sky.

Inside, the room is surprisingly cozy, the lighting warm and inviting. I lay out bowls of water and kibble for Oscar and contemplate what to do next. The fluffy bed beckons, as does the prospect of curling up with a book, but even on a wet day after a three-hundred-mile drive, a new part of me yearns to explore. I remember the brochures: Niagara Falls is only a half hour away and I've never been. I give Oscar a scratch behind the ears, then head to my car.

As I drive to the falls, my expectations lower with each tacky hotel and flashing casino I pass. Crammed parking lots flank the park entrance. By the time I find an empty spot, I'm having doubts about whether I want to stay at all, but I get out and stand in line to purchase a ticket to the *Maid of the Mist,* a tour boat that sails upriver past the base of the American falls and over into the U-shaped basin on the Canadian side. Donning a plastic parka, I board the enormous double-decker ferry with hundreds of other tourists. I have never seen so many selfie sticks in my life.

Squeezing through the crowd, I wedge myself into a decent viewing spot on the lower deck, my ribs pressed up against the starboard railing. Looking around, I can't help but notice I seem to be the only person unaccompanied by family or a significant other. Sightseeing alone, especially in such a crowded setting, makes me self-conscious. "I have friends, I swear," I find myself wanting to tell the couples next to me. Of course, they're too busy admiring the view to notice or to care that I am on my own, but still I feel conspicuous and a bit lonely.

The feeling only lasts a few minutes. As the boat slices through frigid waters, the wind numbs my face and my self-consciousness evaporates amid the onrush of scenery. Instead, my solitude begins to feel luxurious: I can be fully present in a way I couldn't be if traveling with a companion. Flocks of seagulls swoop overhead. As the falls roar into view, the hull of the boat begins to vibrate. What I see before me is infinitely more majestic than anything I could have imagined. Endless gallons of water hurtle over a colossal cliff, smashing, pummeling, and kneading the river into a violent froth. As we approach, freezing water sprays the deck. My parka clings to me like Saran Wrap. Though soaked and shivering, I don't budge. My senses are fully awakened, the world around me too glorious.

It's impossible to confront something so vast and not feel awed. My diagnosis produced a similar effect, and made me wonder how it was I'd ever failed to notice the beauty of my surroundings before or believed that life could be unremarkable. Walking to Mount Sinai for my first round of chemo, knowing it would be my last time out of a hospital room for weeks, I noted every detail, from the shading of the sky to the feel of the breeze on my neck. I thought this new appreciation would stay with me forever, that once I saw, once I knew, how everything could change in an instant, I would never again take such things for granted. But over time, my field of vision narrowed to the size of a ward, then a bed. Walled off from the outside, I had no choice but to turn my gaze inward. Once I was finally released, the threat of imminent death behind me, I only collapsed even further into myself. I stopped paying attention. Here at the foot of the falls, I'm reorienting my gaze outward again.

The next morning, the soft light of a perfect autumn day dapples the dashboard as I ease onto Interstate 90, the northern artery that runs from Boston all the way to Seattle. Between bluffs, I catch glimpses of the vast, royal-blue waters of Lake Erie. Around noon, as I cross over into Pennsylvania's northwestern tip, Oscar begins to whine for a walk. Turning off the highway, I follow the signs to Presque Isle State Park, a thin peninsula that arcs into the lake. Oscar and I stroll along a quiet sandy beach. The lake is enormous—a sea, really—and the shore is fringed with cottonwoods, willows, and oaks. Reflections of golden leaves glimmer like fallen stars on the water.

Much as I've been enjoying my solitude, I find myself wishing Jon were here to share the view. We haven't spoken in a few days, and the distance is already making me feel disconnected from him. Pulling my phone out of my jacket, I dial his number.

"Where y'at?" Jon says, his usual prelude. I can hear the tooting of a trumpet and the belch of a tuba in the background, and I gather that he is rehearsing with the band.

"I'm good," I say, and I'm surprised to realize I actually am. "On my way to Columbus, to visit a man named Howard Crane."

The silence on the end of the line is swollen with words unsaid. When I first told Jon about my plan for a cross-country trip, he made no secret of his disapproval. Though he recognized my need for a drastic change, he didn't like the idea of my traveling alone. He grew even more concerned when he learned I was planning to visit nearly two dozen strangers, most of whom I knew only from the Internet. As Jon pointed out, you can never truly know someone's intentions, no matter how well they present on paper.

"Watch yourself out there," he urges.

I groan, rolling my eyes. "You doing okay?"

"I'm fine. Working nonstop. It's hard not having you here," he says, sounding a little dejected. Right before my departure, Jon had started a new job as the bandleader of a late-night talk show. But just as he'd landed a five-night-a-week gig that allowed him to stop touring and stay in New York, I'd left on my own tour, of sorts. The instruments in the background are growing louder and I'm having trouble making out what he's saying. "Listen, I really want to find a time when we can actually talk. Can I call you after—" Then his voice cuts out.

"You still there?" I ask, even though I know he is gone.

I return to the car deflated. It's not just that we've been out of touch. It's that we've been stuck in a holding pattern. Jon continues to be there for me, hoping I'll eventually be ready to get more serious. But for a whole year, I've been as emotionally available as a bag of rocks. As much as I want to, I don't know how to let him in.

As a kid, I always thought that when you encountered "the one," you experienced a mystical click—a knowing, without a doubt, that this was the person for you. I'd had this conviction in my last relationship, at least at the beginning, but my certainty crumbled with time. "If the relationship ended, it's because it wasn't right for you," a friend reassured me, but the premise still troubles me. What if it was and I just fucked it up?

Over the last year, Jon and I have occasionally broached the topic of a future together. I can entertain it as a fun thought experiment of *what would our kids look like,* but when it comes to actually thinking through the enormity of such a commitment, I panic. Maybe we aren't right for each other. Maybe I'm not capable of being in a relationship with anyone. Maybe it's irresponsible for me to consider long-term vows like marriage or children given my likelihood of relapse.

At the root of it is a deeper uncertainty: Maybe I'll still die.

It's a sort of uncertainty that Howard Crane, the next person on my list, knows well. As I head south through Ohio's Amish country toward his city, the landscape opens, becoming more pastoral, more rolling. I pass a man in suspenders and a straw hat steering a horse and buggy, followed by a second, and a third. Otherwise, the road is empty. To my right and left farmland stretches out beyond what the eye can see. I pick up speed, a cloud of dust gathering around my wheels.

As I approach Columbus, my thoughts turn to Howard's letter, sent three years earlier. An avid reader of *The New York Times,* he'd written me a long response to my first column, "Facing Cancer in Your 20s," which was about the various ways in which age becomes an inextricable component of how we experience illness. *I gather you are by now in the hospital beginning to undergo the bone marrow transplant that will hopefully restore to you the health and well-being most young people take for granted,* he wrote. *I am writing as well because I want to share with you my own experience, which though different in many ways, has nonetheless in its uncertainty and liminality, certain parallels with your own.*

My column had stirred up decades-old memories of his time as a graduate student, in his early thirties, working on archaeological sites in the Sistan Basin in southwest Afghanistan. *As all young people, I thought I was relatively invulnerable, but after two years I suddenly fell ill,* he wrote. *At first I thought I had a form of malaria, but by the third day I realized that it was very unlikely I would make it out of the Sistan. Without going into detail, through a series of what I can only call incomprehensible events, I made my way the 600 miles back to Kabul, and ultimately spent weeks in a hospital in Germany and later in Boston. When I was released, I was physically the likes of an 80 year old man.*

Howard had experienced an array of frightening symptoms— tar-black urine, temporary blindness, and lingering damage to his bone marrow—but, at the time, the doctors were unable to determine a diagnosis. The expectation had been that he wasn't going to survive. *I was so sick that mortality did not frighten me (or perhaps it simply didn't seem real), but in retrospect I have thought about it a great deal,* he wrote. *I know it is a cliché that we should live for the day. And I know it is maybe the hardest thing in the world. We always think ahead, make plans, have hopes. And yet, and yet . . .*

The final lines of his letter left me weeping. *If I believed in the efficacy of prayer, you would be in mine,* he wrote. *Not being a believer, I nonetheless want you to know miracles do abound in this life, that the human body is capable of coping with things that seem insuperable.*

The sun dips low over a row of beige stucco houses with freshly mowed lawns. A mailbox decorated with two cranes tells me I've arrived. I don't get out of the car right away: I need a few minutes to gather myself. I promised Jon that I would do my due diligence before all of my visits, but it's been difficult for me to glean any information about Howard beyond what he shared in the letter. I've found scholarly articles he published in journals and an Ohio State faculty résumé, but he remains nevertheless a total stranger. Steeling myself, I walk up the front path and ring the doorbell.

Howard is tall and thin, with a snowy beard. He stammers a little as he welcomes me inside. I realize he, too, is nervous, which only makes me more so. "Thank you so much for hosting me," I say, following him into the foyer.

"I was absolutely floored when I received your letter," he says. "I never expected to hear from you. So when you said you'd like to visit, it was, for me, something quite extraordinary." Howard is dressed in a black cashmere sweater and a scarf. If his upper half says dignified intellectual, his lower half, with flip-flops and jeans slung low on his hipbones, says child of the sixties.

"My wife, Meral, will be with us soon," he tells me, explaining that she is meeting with a patient in her home office. "In the meantime, let me show you to where you'll be staying."

He leads me down a steep flight of rickety stairs, and when we reach the bottom step, my eyes drift around the basement. It is spacious but crammed full. Hand-painted picket signs protesting the Iraq War. Towering stacks of what appear to be every copy of *The New York Times Magazine* ever published. Wood-paneled walls covered in dozens of newspaper clippings and framed photographs. A half dozen chairs, and a large pullout couch with batik throw pillows where Oscar and I will sleep.

"We're pack rats," Howard says, fluttering his hands around the room, "but I do hope you'll find it comfortable." The basement, he tells me, is where Meral holds support groups for her patients. Howard's entire demeanor changes as he talks about her—the stammer falls away, and his rheumy eyes fill with pride. "She's one of the preeminent therapists for transgender people in the country," he says. "She grew up in Turkey in the forties and fifties, in an environment of much more scarcity than we are familiar with here in America. When she was in primary school, they could only write in pencil so that when they finished an assignment, they could erase it and use their paper over again. These things simply weren't available in Turkey then. Now we live in this plethora of stuff, but she still has a very hard time throwing anything away. I do, too. Clearly!"

As we're speaking, Meral, a striking woman dressed all in black with a leopard-print scarf, descends the steps. She's more assertive and extroverted than Howard, flinging her arms around me, clucking at him for forgetting to offer me a drink. "My Howard has been looking forward to your visit for weeks," she says with a faint trace of an accent. "We both have. Now, shall we go to dinner? You must be starving, poor thing. There's a very nice Turkish restaurant not too far away. Howard will drive."

By the time the appetizers arrive, we have fallen into a good conversational groove. Gracious and inquisitive, Meral and Howard pepper me with questions. They are pleased to discover that I, too, have spent time in the Middle East. I tell them about studying abroad in Egypt, about my research on women's rights in postcolonial North Africa, and about my family in Tunisia. People rarely ask about my pre-illness interests, and as I recount long-forgotten pastimes, I feel as though I am touring someone else's life.

There's an old Tunisian saying that your entire life is inscribed on your forehead but it's as though everything that came before my diagnosis has been scrubbed from mine. I don't know how it happened, or if it could have been prevented, but at some point in the last few years my entire existence, my identity, even my career, became linked to the worst thing that ever happened to me. My scope of interests shrank in direct proportion to my world. A year out of treatment, illness continues to dominate the narrative and seems to squeeze out the possibilities of anything else.

The next morning, I join Meral and Howard in the living room. We lounge around on the couch and watch the news. Their cat, an old tabby, curls up on Howard's lap. As political pundits discuss the Obama administration's decision to keep troops in Afghanistan, Howard scowls, tsking and grumbling that the world is going to hell. "Time to write another op-ed," he says.

"Have you always been a big letter writer?" I ask.

"I guess you could call it my hobby," he says. He tells me that he first started writing letters when he met Meral. They were apart for the first two years of their relationship—she was just out of high school and living in Berkeley; he was attending college three thousand miles away in Cambridge. "Telephoning cost an arm and a leg and we didn't have the money to do those sorts of things. A three-cent postage letter was about what we could afford."

"Each of us wrote a letter a day," Meral chimes in. "Sometimes two letters a day."

"I don't know how we filled them up," Howard says, shaking his head in wonder. "One day I got a letter from her that was twenty-seven pages long! What could possibly have happened in twenty-four hours to fill twenty-seven pages?"

Howard and Meral had continued letter writing over the years whenever they were apart, including during his days in Afghanistan. From a hospital bed in Kabul, a young Howard had dictated what he believed to be a last letter to Meral, expecting never to see her again. In fact, he went on to make an astounding recovery, but it wasn't the last time he would find himself grappling with mortality. Eventually, doctors diagnosed him with common variable immunodeficiency. He, like me, suffers from a compromised immune system, and over the last decades has experienced an uninterrupted chain of infections, some of them life-threatening. But Howard, unlike me, hasn't allowed any of it to keep him from loving and being loved. He hasn't just embraced uncertainty, he's constructed a whole life inside of it, building and rebuilding as many times as has been necessary. In spite of his health, he got married, had two kids, and pursued a career that he found infinitely fascinating.

It has not been without difficulties, of course. He tells me about receiving a prestigious appointment as chair of the art history department at Ohio State, only to step down five years later because he was so unwell. And yet, Howard persisted in finding workarounds for his limitations. "Winter was the worst season for me," Howard said, explaining that he would frequently get pneumonia. "I had to hibernate, so I started teaching only in the warmer months."

Howard is retired, but spends his days reading, taking long walks in the nearby park, and firing off an occasional letter to the editor. He and Meral are grandparents now. They recently celebrated their fiftieth wedding anniversary. And once a week they take ballroom dancing classes together.

When I ask if he has guidance for me, he deflects, telling me to ask Meral, the therapist, instead. "She's quite directive," he says. "She doesn't believe in people magically finding their own way, because they often don't. They end up spending years—shall I use a cuss word?—*mindfucking*," he says, with a giggle.

"Come on, I'm not letting you off that easily," I press.

A moment passes, and Howard relents. "Slowly, with enough patience and persistence, you'll become immersed in life again and, let's face it, life can be so good. But I think it's most important to find someone who has the wherewithal to stick it out with you. I owe more to my wife—" His voice catches. "Well, what I owe her, it's beyond expression."

"Sounds like I need to find myself a Meral," I say.

Seeing them together makes me want to open myself up to the future, but hard as I try, I still can't imagine myself growing old, alone or with anyone else. To learn to swim in the ocean of not-knowing—this is my constant work. I can't know if there is a rogue cancer cell lurking somewhere in my marrow. I can't predict if my body will scuttle commitments to myself or to others. I'm not even sure I want to settle down in a stable, more conventional way. But I'm beginning to understand this: We never know. Life is a foray into mystery.

30

WRITTEN ON THE SKIN

IT'S EARLY MORNING in Eastern Market, an industrial neighborhood in Detroit. I'm staying with Nitasha, a young woman in her early thirties with long black curls and a witchy, ethereal quality. A digital marketer for a pharmacy by day, artist by night, and Frida Kahlo aficionada at all hours, she's hosting me in a large open loft with twenty-foot ceilings and brick walls covered in her paintings. When I arrived last night, she was simmering homemade harissa on the stove in honor of my Tunisian heritage. As we tore off chunks of bread and dipped them into the spicy chili paste, she told me that she'd first learned of me years earlier, through following Melissa online. "I saw a portrait she painted of you and was so moved by your friendship," she said. Partially inspired by our struggles, she's working on a plan to use her loft as an exhibition space for what she's calling "The Museum of Healing." It will showcase works by local artists exploring topics related to disease, medicine, and recovery.

Our first stop this morning is the farmers market, only a few blocks away. Nitasha leads me through open-air stalls selling mason jars of pickles, luscious heads of lettuce, and artisanal soaps made of goat milk. As we wander, she tells me about dermatographism, a skin condition she's lived with since she was eight. She, too, knows what it's like to be plagued by an itch: "Itching and itching. And even more itching," she says, "until I wish I could unzip my own skin!" Even the most minor scratches morph into welts that last a half hour.

But Nitasha, like Frida Kahlo, has turned her predicament into art. She traces a few arcs idly on her forearm with a fingernail and I watch as they thicken into red icing. She says she draws on her skin this way—sometimes making detailed geometric patterns, sometimes written messages—then culls inspiration from the results. In one installation piece called *Skin Suit*, she experimented with leaving rusty objects on fabric, and layered the stains to create patterns, mimicking the appearance of skin under a magnifying glass. "I see my body as an extension of my sketchbook," she tells me as we exit the hipster market and begin wandering along the vacant streets, passing warehouses and abandoned buildings. "It also comes in handy for writing down phone numbers," she adds, laughing.

Later that afternoon, Nitasha takes me for a drive around the city. We pass an abandoned house where a tree's branches have begun sprouting through its walls. We come across vacant lots that urban farmers have turned into homesteads of organic produce. We meander along the sidewalks of the Heidelberg Project, a neighborhood where neglected homes have been transformed into public art pieces painted in psychedelic polka dots with lawn sculptures made from mounds of dolls and other found objects. We stop in front of the brick façade of a warehouse, spray-painted in clouds of tangerine and aquamarine blue. On the bottom right-hand corner, there is an inscription by the artist Fel3000ft that reads like a rallying cry for rebuilding from any catastrophe:

*We have been considered many things: A city in decay, a
city in distress and without hope. However, we have never
given up and we never say die. We are born fighters, we rise
from the ashes. We are a community that believes in our
future despite whatever anyone throws against us. We are
Detroit!*

I am learning to read the moods of cities, and perhaps more
than anywhere else so far, I relate to Detroit, a city of many narratives. A place powered by the auto industry that powered America.
A place inscribed by segregation, but also by such promise that
tens of thousands of black Americans settled there during the
Great Migration. A place that nearly died when the car companies
downsized and left, but didn't die, refuses to die. A place where the
future is painted upon the palimpsest of a painful past. Upon skin
that rears up in welts, angry and beautiful—a beauty that tran-
scends anger but also wouldn't be possible without it. And isn't
that how it always goes, catastrophe forcing reinvention?

Before I leave Detroit, Nitasha takes me to one more place: a psychic's storefront with a sign in the window advertising tarot card
and tea leaf readings. She insists this psychic is not a fraud but a
true clairvoyant whose specialty is in healing damaged souls. I've
never done anything like this before, and the logical part of me
thinks it's a waste. But the part of me that wants to dispel the uncertainty in my life—to conjure the illusion of knowing what's
going to happen to me—can't resist.

Behind the modest storefront is an incense-fogged room lined
with shelves of crystals, oils, and herbs for sale. The psychic, a
young man dressed in a skintight, rhinestone-encrusted T-shirt
and acid-washed jeans, leads me to the back. Behind a heavy curtain, we sit facing each other, my hands in his hands, our faces
bathed in the flickering light of votive candles. Over the next few

minutes, his body begins to shake and his eyes roll into the back of his head, seized by what I can only assume are "visions." I look on skeptically, already regretting the crisp fifty I'll have to fork over at the end of this.

When the psychic opens his eyes, he tells me he's been visited by an ancestor—a woman, perhaps an aunt, on the paternal side of my family. He tilts his head back as if to take a long sip of water, lips opening and closing, eyelids twitching with the ferocity of a man possessed. When he reopens his eyes he tells me this aunt of mine was very sick before she died. Then he asks if I, too, have been sick.

I try to maintain my cool as I reply that, yes, I've been sick, and that, yes, now that I think of it, my father had a sister, Gmar, who died very young of a mysterious illness. He tells me that Gmar has spent many nights and days worrying for me and has done her best to keep me safe. Although my body is clear of danger I am on a different kind of odyssey now—a long, arduous one that will take me deep into the unknown before I will find clarity. As he speaks, goosebumps erupt on my arms. For a moment, I wonder, *Did I give him my name? Any other information? Is it my short hair that tipped him off?* I don't think so, but it doesn't matter to me anymore. Leaning forward in my chair, I want to know more.

The psychic spreads a deck of tarot cards onto the table and invites me to choose. With each card I draw, he sees deeper into me. I will write a book, one that will take me all over the world, he claims. He sees that it will be a struggle for me to commit to a partner, but that, after a long spell of uncertainty, I'll eventually settle down with a woman—wait, no, a man, he corrects—and then he mutters a bunch of incantations.

I know the psychic is probably telling me what he thinks I want to hear, but I envision my future as a long corridor of closed doors, and with each of his predictions, a door opens and I can see farther ahead. Until now, time for me has been measured in short increments—the biopsy up ahead, the doctor's appointment on the horizon. Imagining a future is a frightening exercise when your life has been upended; it requires hope, which feels risky, even dangerous. But as the psychic speaks, as he tells me of the long, expansive life that I'm destined to lead, as he presents my future as an inevitability, it starts to seem possible.

"What else?" I ask the psychic, my face open, gullible.

The next day, rain drizzles through the bare trees. The sky is a matte gray, the air wet and heavy. In past cities, I've always taken bad weather as an omen that it's time to continue on—and it's true, I'm due to go. But even in the chill, with my heater cranked up as the rain spatters the windshield, I find it hard to leave Detroit.

On the road, while thinking about my next stop, my mind flits back to my fourth and final hospital stay for *C. diff*. Though it's only been a year, I can't recall much of anything—I've tried to erase those last days in treatment and with Will. But what I remember most clearly is that I felt an overpowering instinct to self-isolate, like a wounded coyote who deserts its pack when it senses the end is near. With the knowledge that Will was preparing to move out of our apartment, I couldn't stay stoic. I sent my mother home and accepted no visitors. I told everyone I was fine, when in fact I needed the privacy to fall apart.

Bret, whom I'm on my way to see now, was an exception to the no-visitors rule during that period. He was the one who approached me in the waiting room of the transplant clinic, recognizing me from the column. I remember thinking how fortuitous it was that we had ended up seated next to each other that day; it was my first time going to chemo alone, his first time at Sloan Kettering, and the presence of another young patient comforted us both. After that day, we stayed in touch, exchanging occasional emails, phone calls, and medical advice. We only met once more, but in some ways I felt closer and more connected to him than I did to my family and friends. Trauma has a way of dividing your view of the world into two camps: those who get it and those who don't.

The last time we saw each other, Bret was about to embark on a road trip of his own. His doctors had declared him stable enough to transfer his care to a hospital closer to home, and he and his wife, Aura, were heading back to Chicago. Before leaving for good, the two of them burst through my hospital room door, giddy with possibility. They brought me a silly hat from a gas station— a white beret with glittery netting and glue-on crystals that looked absurd over my short hair. It made me profoundly happy to see Bret doing well, and I took an instant liking to Aura, whose radiance filled the room and, from everything I'd heard, deserved a gold medal in caregiving. I was cheered by their visit, but after they left, I felt down again. Seeing them—so happy together in spite of everything they'd been through—was proof that it was possible for love to survive a prolonged illness. It showed me how things could have worked out differently for me and Will, and raised painful questions about why they didn't.

On the South Side of Chicago, I pull up to a wood-shingled Victorian located in a quiet neighborhood. Bret gives me a tour, telling me they stretched their budget a year earlier to buy this place, their first home. He's been trying to keep busy with little renovation projects; he just finished fixing a leak in the roof. They're hoping for a baby sometime in the near future, he says, but there's still a lot of work to be done. I admire the hardwood floors and the big bay windows in the living room, the sunlit dining room, and the study, which he tells me they have plans to turn into a nursery. The *adultness* of it all impresses me—the way they drink gourmet coffee on the back porch, keep houseplants alive, pay a mortgage. They are in their early thirties, just a few years older than me, but their lives seem so much more sophisticated, the opposite of sleeping in campgrounds and on couches, subsisting on gas station coffee and peanut butter and jelly sandwiches.

Aura is a public school social worker, and she's still at work. Bret tells me about how committed she is to her students, many of whom live in dangerous, low-income neighborhoods. What free time she has, when she isn't helping care for her husband, is dedicated to organizing education reform initiatives and protests. "My wife works so fucking hard," Bret says. "The least I can do is to make sure she comes home to a beautiful home and a nice meal." He gets to work making a cashew-chicken curry, uncorking a bottle of wine, and setting the table for dinner.

From the outside, it is easy to assume Bret and Aura lead a charmed life, but when the three of us sit down to eat, they catch me up on the events of the last year, which include a near-fatal heart attack Bret recently suffered, likely caused by blood vessel damage from the radiation he received during treatment. Bret also has GVHD, which we've both struggled with. My case has thankfully been mild and remains under control, except for a rash that sometimes flares on my forehead. His, however, has noticeably worsened since we last saw each other, attacking his lungs and leaving his eyes and skin a violent red.

A filmmaker before, Bret is now on disability. His hands shake from the immunosuppressants, so he can't hold a camera steady. It isn't clear when or if he will ever be well enough to return to work. For the foreseeable future he must depend on his wife to take care of him—not only physically, but financially as well. Without health insurance through her job, he would not survive. "I've been the recipient of so much support and love and I want desperately to contribute to the world, but I can't," he says, his tone suddenly somber.

Though rid of the lymphoma that once plagued his body, Bret is, in many ways, sicker than he's ever been. "I'm two years out of transplant, and I still feel like hell," he confesses as we wash dishes after dinner. "My hands ache, my muscles and joints wake me up at five in the morning. And I can't close the lid on my pillbox because there's so much medication in there." This is the cruel irony of medicine: Sometimes the treatments you receive to get better make you worse in the long run, requiring further care, exposing you to yet more complications and side effects. It is a maddening cycle.

"I made it through the transplant, I made it through the heart attack, and I'm so fucking lucky to be alive," Bret says to me the next afternoon. Rain pelts the windows. We're listening to Tina Turner on the record player. Oscar and Hodge, their golden retriever–corgi mix, are curled up between us on the couch. "But each time something happens, it's a little bit harder to come back, you know?"

I nod and murmur yes in agreement, and he continues. "It's like the late rounds of a boxing match," he says. "You're beyond tired and you know that things are probably only going to get worse and yet you have to find some way to keep fighting. But sometimes I can't help but wonder, *What's the point?* So many people get better, then get something deadlier. You had lymphoma and it comes back as leukemia. Your liver's so overloaded with toxins it's gonna jump ship any day now."

"Skin cancer coming down the road, guaranteed!" I jump in, and we both laugh.

Bret and I have both learned the hard way to brace ourselves for bad news; our bodies and thus our lives are capable of implosion at a moment's notice. In a way, setbacks were easier to deal with when we were still in treatment: We were prepared for the possibility that things could take a turn. But when the body betrays you again and again, it obliterates whatever nascent trust you've restored in the universe and your place in it. Each time, it becomes harder to recover your sense of safety. After you've had the ceiling cave in on you—whether through illness or some other catastrophe—you don't assume structural stability. You must learn to live on fault lines.

That night, I begin to think about how porous the border is between the sick and the well. It's not just people like Bret and me who exist in the wilderness of survivorship. As we live longer and longer, the vast majority of us will travel back and forth across these realms, spending much of our lives somewhere in between. These are the terms of our existence. The idea of striving for some beautiful, perfect state of wellness? It mires us in eternal dissatisfaction, a goal forever out of reach.

To be well now is to learn to accept whatever body and mind I currently have.

31

THE VALUE OF PAIN

THE WAY WE heal does not always look like healing. When I left home forty days ago, I envisioned the road trip as an opportunity to start living again. I thought the farther I drove, the farther I'd get from the hospital hallways I floated down in a cotton gown, mumbling to myself, high on morphine; the farther I'd feel from the room at the Hope Lodge where I waited up in bed for Will, with a cold dread welling in my gut; the farther I'd be from the matchbox apartment on Avenue A where we made a home—and then bulldozed it.

Move on already, I tell myself. *Get over it!* But the more mileage I put between Will and me, the more preoccupied I become by what happened to us. The unraveling of our relationship seems worse to me after seeing Bret and Aura find a way to thrive together, even plan for a baby, despite the ongoingness of his health struggles.

Everywhere I look these days I see ghosts of Will. Silhouettes of sapling-tall men with square jaws and floppy hair that make my pulse scamper. I wonder, irrationally, if that could really be him sitting at the Formica counter of a mom-and-pop diner in rural Iowa, wolfing down chicken fingers and french fries, or trout fishing on the grassy banks of a river in the Sandhills of Nebraska, where I spent a weekend camping. These apparitions are mostly in my head, but on some days, someone or something invokes his name unexpectedly, and the hidden parts of the past that live inside me rise up to my eyes, an eddying, swirling flood of regret and rage, until I can see nothing else. I've spent so much time trying to bury the memory of him, and of us, that a reckoning seems unavoidable.

I am driving through Pine Ridge, one of the poorest Native American reservations in the country, as tumbleweeds scrape along the road. The land is stark and scrubbed. The air is steeped in a stillness that settles around everything like sediment—the pop-up trailers, the shacks made of scrap wood and tarp, the rusted piles of dismembered cars. The night before, I crashed on the living room floor of a ponytailed motorcyclist in Lead, South Dakota. He used to work on this reservation and said it was worth stopping by for a visit. Before I left, he had put me in touch with the staff of Thunder Valley, a community regeneration project on "the rez"—as he and everyone around here call it.

In the vacant parking lot of Thunder Valley, the wind hisses and howls, the cold stinging my face like a slap. I'm met by a young man, a citizen of the Oglala Lakota nation, who introduces himself as the founding director of this place. He's burly and baby-faced with tawny skin covered in tattoos and a glossy black braid that snakes down his back. "Nick," he says, giving me a firm handshake and leading me into one of the double-wides that constitute Thunder Valley's headquarters.

We take a seat at a table and Nick begins to tell me about the work they do here. I'm interested in all of it—the sustainable housing pilot project using a straw-bale building technique, the community garden to help ameliorate the shortage of fresh food on the reservation—but I can't seem to focus. Something about Nick is familiar, this whole place is familiar, and the synapses in my brain crackle distractingly.

"Have we met before?" I interrupt.

"I was just wondering the same thing," he says. "What'd you say your name was again?"

I repeat my name, first and last, articulating the slew of vowels more slowly.

Leaning forward a little in our seats, we stare at each other, trying to locate some long-forgotten folder in the filing cabinets of memory. And then it clicks. "Will," we both say.

It still seems unbelievable. I've been trying so hard to block out the past that I've come all the way here—to Pine Ridge, to Thunder Valley, to meet Nick—without connecting any of the dots: Will's father, a documentary filmmaker and reporter, had covered the reservation early on in his career. He'd told me about how, in the late sixties, the Native Americans, fed up with centuries of mistreatment by the federal government, had organized a grassroots effort known as the American Indian Movement and led protests across the country, one of which had culminated in a deadly shootout with two FBI agents at Pine Ridge in 1975. Will's father was the only non–Native American journalist present during the shootings. He'd been outside Jumping Bull, a ranch on the southwest corner of the rez, when some of the bullets went flying. A stray round hit his pickup, and he'd crouched low behind the truck with a portable tape deck, recording it all for an NPR broadcast.

In my early days in Paris, when Will and I were in the pen pal phase, he had told me about accompanying his father on reporting trips as a kid, which was where he'd befriended Nick and his family. He had even sent me an article about Nick's work at Thunder Valley. *If you ever plan to be in the US for more than a week, we could go visit,* he wrote. *It's a part of the country few people ever see.* Still in the tentative stages of courtship, I remember being far less interested in the Thunder Valley article than in deciphering Will's usage of *we,* which had left me hopeful that he also saw this as a relationship that might continue off the page.

Both Nick and I keep shaking our heads as we piece this all together, utterly dumbfounded by the strangeness of meeting here, today, under entirely unrelated circumstances. He's heard all about me from Will—about my illness, about my writing—and it turns out I'm even Facebook friends with his sister.

"What a small world," Nick marvels.

"What a small world," I echo, less marveling than disturbed by all that I've blotted out.

"How's Will doing anyway?" he asks. "It's been a minute since we caught up."

My shoulders slump when I realize Nick doesn't know. I still have no idea how to tell the story of what happened to Will and me and whenever I try, I can hear the venom creeping into my voice despite my best efforts to keep it at bay. I know it isn't fair to make Will out to be the villain—it doesn't account for the countless ways in which he loved me, stood by me, fought to stay—but I'm still unable to narrate it any other way.

"I'm not sure what he's up to these days," I finally say, trying to keep my voice steady, but the anger is there, quivering right below the surface.

"Oh," Nick says. "I had no idea you two split. Man, I'm so sorry."

"I'm sorry, too." I mop my eyes with the back of my arm once, hard, before changing the topic. These wiped western skies are too big, the aperture blasted too far open: It all makes me feel overexposed. In extremis, you feel like this, peeled back and vulnerable to the world.

I spend the night on the reservation at a motel called the Lakota Prairie Ranch Resort. My room overlooks a parking lot and has a sticky carpet and fraying bedspread. On the bathroom counter I find a small pile of oil-stained towels next to a laminated card that reads: "For your convenience: PLEASE use these rags to clean spills, shoes, guns."

I throw the bedspread on the floor, unfurl my sleeping bag over the mattress, and spend the next few hours trying to convince myself I am asleep when, in fact, I am thinking about Will. I remember how, after my diagnosis, Nick had invited Will to bring me to Pine Ridge for a healing ceremony called a Sun Dance. How, when my doctors told me I wasn't well enough to travel, Will had decided to go to Pine Ridge without me. How it made me angry whenever Will traveled without me. The fact that he could go places and I couldn't had highlighted the difference between me and him—between me and my peers, between me and all the able-bodied people of the world. I still couldn't make sense of why some people suffered and others did not, why some lives were heaped in misfortune while others were spared. To be young and sick was unfair, so much so that it had felt unbearable in moments. I had always understood, at least in theory, that to rage against all this was pointless—poisonous. But still, I compared my limitations to the liberties of others. I wanted their freedom so badly that I hated them for it.

Behind my closed eyelids, a fire of remorse blazes, keeping me awake. While it's easy to destroy the past, it's far more difficult to forget it. My mind keeps replaying the first big fight Will and I ever had. Like so many first fights, it contained the seeds of dissent that would later blossom much larger. We were supposed to be traveling to Santa Barbara in a few days to celebrate the wedding of one of Will's childhood friends. We hadn't boarded a plane since I'd started treatment, and I was looking forward to a change of scenery. But as the departure date approached it became clear that unless my blood counts miraculously improved, I wouldn't be able to go. Up until the last minute, however, I kept insisting that I was well enough.

My desperation to participate in the world often clouded my judgment, meaning Will regularly had to take on the unpleasant role of enforcer. And a few nights before we were supposed to leave, he sat me down. "I talked it over with your parents," Will said gently, putting an arm around my shoulder and pulling me into him. "You know how much I want you to come, but we all agree: It's just not safe for you to get on a plane right now. You need to stay home and rest."

I remember being overwhelmed by a desire to scream, my rage so great I wanted to reach up and rip down the sky. Will was right—boarding a plane in my condition was a death wish. I knew he was just trying to look out for me, but I didn't know where else to direct my anger. Jerking away from him, I said, "How *dare* you convene with my parents behind my back. Like I'm some child incapable of making decisions for myself. Like I don't feel pathetic enough. And let me guess—you're going to go without me."

I watched this man—who had not been home to see his family or friends in months, who had not left my side since the diagnosis, who had spent a summer of sleepless nights on a cot next to my hospital bed—crumple. "Sus," he pleaded, "please don't be upset. I just need a break."

"Yeah? Well, I need one, too," I snapped back.

The next day, I woke up smarting with shame. I knew better. I understood how important it is for caregivers to be granted the gift of guilt-free time to themselves. Will both deserved and desperately needed a break, and I told myself that just because I was too sick to go didn't mean he should have to stay home, too. With this in mind, I tried to stow my anger when Will left for the wedding. But it was hard to keep down for long. No matter how deeply buried, it found its way out.

As pictures of Will's trip filtered onto my Facebook timeline over the next few days, I began to smolder. With each new picture I saw—Will and his friends hanging out at the beach, playing soccer, at a bar, dancing—my anger bubbled closer to the surface. Alone in my bedroom, the irrational part of me took over: Maybe Will was secretly relieved that I hadn't been well enough to join him. Without my being there, he could go out as late as he wanted. A sick girlfriend was a liability, a buzzkill, always threatening to ruin the party or cut short the night because she was tired yet again.

Of course, I was really raging at the dismal blood counts that had prevented me from accompanying him, at the body that kept me bound to bed, at the chemo I would have to do later that week, at the possibility that my life was over before it had really begun. But it is hard to rage at something as nebulous as cancer. You have to steer the trajectory of your anger, ideally toward a canvas or a notebook, before it hurtles toward a human target—but I didn't know how to do this then. When Will called from the wedding after-party, sounding goofy and carefree and a little buzzed, I found a pretext to pick a fight. All weekend I did this, berating him for all kinds of ridiculous things—not calling right when he said he would, not responding to a text quickly enough.

At the core of my anger was a fear that while spending time out there, in the world, Will would realize all that he was missing. Fear that he would grow weary of having to take care of me, that he would leave and would not return.

What I wish I'd known then: Untamed fear consumes you, becomes you, until what you are most afraid of turns alive.

Toward the end of Will's trip, I spiked a high fever and went back to the hospital, where I was admitted for what would end up being a multi-week stay. Will got on the next flight and came straight from the airport to the cancer ward, where he found me tied up to tubes and machines, my breathing labored, my face ashen, yet another infection spreading through my blood. Sitting at my bedside, he bowed his head in his hands and wept. "I never should have gone," he said.

A confession: In that moment, I was secretly pleased to have gotten so sick while he was away. It meant he was forced to cut his trip short. It meant he was back in the Bubble with me and that I wasn't as alone. It meant he would think twice about leaving again. I really believed that if I could keep him close, it would keep us from growing apart. I was so young.

Before leaving Pine Ridge, I read up on the Sun Dance, a centuries-old sacred healing ceremony that takes place each summer. It begins with a team of more than a hundred men working together to cut down a towering tree in a nearby forest. Using a complex set of harnesses, they lower it, being careful to keep the tree from touching the forest floor, then load it onto a flatbed. Once the tree has been safely transported back to the reservation, the men hoist it into the center of a circular outdoor arena nested in a gap between the mountains known as Thunder Valley.

The tree is the physical and spiritual centerpiece of the ceremony. Its branches are adorned with hundreds of "tobacco ties," offerings of tobacco leaf wrapped in multicolored cloths, each hue signifying a different prayer. The men pierce their skin with needles and attach ropes from their chests to the trunk. Forsaking all food and drinking only a small amount of water, they sing and dance and pray for four days straight in the blistering sun, many of them collapsing to the ground. Pain, heat, dehydration, and hunger aren't unfortunate perils: They are part of the process. The dancers believe that by simulating death, they alleviate the pain and sorrows of both their community and their ancestors. It's not about penance or the glorification of suffering, but about re-creating and honoring the cycle of life and death. Following a final purification ritual, they are meant to reenter the world anew, spiritually cleansed and fortified for what lies ahead.

It's a lesson in the value of pain.

I'm realizing that if I am to cross the distance between near-death and renewal, instead of trying to bury my pain, I must use it as a guide to know myself better. In confronting my past, I have to reckon not only with the pain of losing other people but also with the pain I've caused others. I must keep seeking truths and teachers on these long, lonely stretches of highway even when—especially when—the search brings discomfort.

Somewhere between South Dakota and Wyoming, the fall chill turns to killing frost and the trees empty of birds. I roll down a window and stick a hand out, and my fingers quickly go numb. A wet, chalky scent fills the air. It starts to snow, a flake falling here, a flake falling there, and my mind begins to wander. As I travel the land in between, it feels at times as though all I am is memory. I rewind old scenes from my life, seeing countless mistakes and regrettable choices, unable to do anything about them now except better understand what happened.

In this particular moment, I find myself midway through a memory of a phone conversation I had with my father toward the end of that final hospital stay. I had just announced to him that Will was moving out and that I didn't think we would be getting back together. "You are my daughter and I love you more than anyone," my father told me. "But I'm not sure that at Will's age I would have been capable of being there for you in the way he has."

I remember feeling hurt after we hung up. Instead of lauding Will, he should have been upset with him for leaving me. At the time, I was still too angry to understand what my father really meant. As I drive, I'm still trying to make sense of it.

In my mind, I've forgiven Will for moving out, but in my heart, I still feel betrayed. Will and I don't speak but occasionally he'll email or text me a random picture—a handwritten list of my chemo medications with instructions he jotted down in a journal, a photograph of me lying on a gurney with an oxygen mask strapped to my face. I can't tell if he's doing it out of nostalgia or hostility—his way of saying, *Look at all I did for you.* I hate the way these missives remind me of how much I needed him, and remind me of the hold he still has on me. Just thinking about it makes me furious. "Fuck you, fuck you, fuck you," I sing as I drive. I want him to stop blaming me for his troubles. I want him to apologize for the ways he hurt me—then I can finally stop being angry, I tell myself.

The Tetons serrate the horizon. I merge onto the John D. Rockefeller Jr. Memorial Parkway, a majestic stretch of highway that leads to Yellowstone National Park, but I'm too absorbed in thought to admire my surroundings. It occurs to me that at twenty-seven I'm now the same age Will was when I got sick. At the time, the five-year age difference between us had seemed colossal in the way that it does when you're twenty-two and each year of life might as well be a decade. *Mon vieux,* I'd once jokingly called Will when we were living in Paris.

As I drive through what has become a swirling mist of snow, I try to imagine what I would do if I found myself in Will's position now. I try to imagine being there for someone I've only been dating for a few months who has just received a deadly diagnosis. I try to imagine packing my bags, flying to a small town I've never visited before, and moving in with his parents; spending months of my life sleeping on a hospital cot; turning down promotions at work at a time when most of my friends are focused on building their careers. I try to imagine how I would cope with being the receptacle of his anger. I try to imagine shopping for an engagement ring all the while knowing that the one I love may not survive.

When I try to imagine myself doing all of this, I flounder. I can't. I doubt I would be capable of doing a fraction of what Will did for me.

The truth is, I couldn't hear Will's needs above the clamor of my own. I needed constant reassurance that my needs weren't too much. When my needs did become too much, I made it impossible for him to take the breaks he so desperately needed. In those final months, whenever he accompanied me on yet another trip to the emergency room, the look on his face had been one of exhausted obligation. I took this as evidence that I was indeed a burden, and that he was biding his time until he could finally leave. But in the end, it wasn't the illness that had driven him away; it was me. It was the countless little ways in which I'd been pushing him away for years, daring him to go until, one day, he finally did.

I'm so sorry, I whisper into the dark.

It's snowing harder now, and my windshield wipers are working overtime. I think about calling it a night and finding a motel until the storm calms, but I worry that the more I delay this leg of my journey west, the worse the driving conditions will become. I decide to continue on until I hit the Montana state line. With no other cars in sight, my tires leave tracks in the fresh, unspoiled powder. The ponderosa pines flanking the highway sag under the weight of the snow, their branches dripping with icicles, everything twinkling in that chilled, bluest light.

Over the next hour, what's left of my anger at Will drains away. In its place, I am able to feel what anger hasn't allowed me to feel, and there is so much I want to say. Will may not have been there for me at the end, but he was there for me when it counted. I want to ask him for forgiveness. I want to tell him how much I miss him.

If this were a movie, I would call Will from the road right now. Maybe, we'd even find our way back to each other. But this is not a movie. Last we spoke, Will had gotten a new job as an editor heading up a sports site. I've heard he's dating someone new and that the two of them are happy. To love Will now is to appreciate memories of us, without allowing myself to be seduced by their siren call. It's to resist picking up the phone. It's to give him the space he needs to reclaim his life. It's to do what's hardest. To let him go.

As I near the Montana border, I pass through a side-of-the-highway, blink-and-you-miss-it kind of town. The main road is empty, except for a lone car trailing behind me. Over the next few blocks, the car scoots up until it is following at an uncomfortably close distance. Through the snow, a beam of red light swirls from its roof but I'm too wrapped up in my thoughts to notice. It's only when I hear the beep-beep warning of a siren that I finally register I am being tailed by a police car.

I've never been pulled over, and my old driving instructor, Brian, failed to cover this in our lessons. Flustered, I swerve over to the side of the road and park, and in a deeply misguided attempt to show compliance, I open the door, thinking I'll meet the police officer midway between our two cars. But as soon as my boot touches the frozen ground, I understand I've committed a grave error—an error that, for people who don't look like me or have my privileges, could be a matter of life or death.

"Get back in the vehicle!" the officer shouts. "GET. BACK. IN. THE. VEHICLE."

Terrified, I duck into the car, slamming the door shut. Oscar is barking loudly and I'm hissing at him to shut up when the officer appears, rapping his gloved knuckles on the window.

"I'm sorry," I say as the glass lowers. "I thought I was supposed to meet you outside the car. I thought it was the polite thing to do," I explain idiotically, panting a little.

The officer has a spray of pimples across his cheeks and looks boyish, but the expression on his face isn't exactly friendly. "Don't ever do that again," he says, staring me down. "Do you know why I pulled you over?"

"No, sir."

"You were going five miles over the speed limit."

I open my mouth to apologize again, but the officer holds up his palm, silencing me. "License and registration."

I fumble through the glove compartment, which is stuffed full of crap—maps, odd papers, ChapStick, and, inexplicably, a child's Slinky.

"That's it right there," the officer says, pointing.

A few minutes later the officer returns with my license and registration, peering down at me through the open window. He's got a few more questions, starting with how it is that, as a new driver, I've ended up in Wyoming with a vehicle that has New York license plates, and why it is registered in someone else's name.

"Actually, it's a funny story," I say, launching into a rambling explanation about cancer and kingdoms, a one-hundred-day road trip, and my friend who lent me the car. I'm revved with adrenaline and it's hard to tell if I'm making any sense.

"All right, miss. Calm down," he says. The corners of his mouth twitch as he suppresses a smile. "I'm going to let you off with a warning," he says. "But lemme get this straight. You're a new driver. You've borrowed your friend's car. You're on a road trip."

I nod as he says each phrase.

"But why in the name of all that's good and holy are you driving in the middle of a blizzard?"

32

SALSA AND
THE SURVIVALISTS

AS I TRAVEL deeper into the wilderness of Montana, I see no one on the road for miles and miles. The land is immense and veiled in knee-deep snow, the sky so vast it makes me feel like the only person in the world. I've been driving in silence for several hours when my phone rings. I jump, a bit startled. I glance over and see Jon's name flash across the screen; I let it go to voicemail. I've had so much on my mind lately that I don't know how to share with him. When we do speak these days, our conversations are little more than strained chitchat. Have we run out of things to say? With half a continent's distance between us, it's hard to remember what makes us good together. The future of our relationship was always somewhat precarious, and what's between us seems increasingly unlikely to survive the trip.

Loss has left me guarded, spent, and not just the loss of life I've witnessed over the last few years. It's the collateral losses of illness: of Will, of fertility and motherhood as I'd envisioned it, of my identity and my footing in this world. At times, my heart feels so haunted that there's no room for the living—for the possibility of new love, new loss.

Just last night, I received a message from someone I care about that sent me into a deep and guarded retreat. After driving all day in the blizzard, I checked into a bed-and-breakfast in Gardiner, Montana, and decided to take a bath in the claw-foot tub to thaw out and decompress. I filled the tub until it was almost brimming, removed my boots and wool socks and stripped off the rest of my clothes. Submerging my body into the hot water, I sighed as every muscle slackened. After soaking for a while, I reached over the edge of the tub and picked up my phone with slippery fingers. Since being on the road, I'd let a stack of emails pile up in my in-box, and I figured I should get caught up.

Skimming the dozens of unread messages, I saw one from my friend Max; he'd sent it a week and a half earlier. The subject line—*Health Update*—made me tense up. Lots of patients send mass emails to keep friends and family in the loop—these sorts of messages don't always contain bad news. But in the four years I'd known him, Max had never sent a mass health update before. I knew that whatever news this email contained wouldn't be good.

I stared at my phone for a while, then put it down on the tiled floor. I didn't want to read the message, to step through that door. I slipped my head underwater, then opened my eyes and watched little air bubbles escape from my lips and rise to the surface. I bobbed back up, the water sloshing around me. Once the surface had stilled, I picked up my phone again and began to read.

Dear All,

My cancer is back in my lungs and throat, and I'm going to undergo surgery tomorrow at Cedars Sinai in Los Angeles. The recovery time on this surgery is unknown—we don't know how difficult the tumors will be to access. We also don't know at this moment if the immune treatment I was on was effective in some measure, or if it wasn't effective at all. The surgery will determine all of this, and help us plan next steps.

If you need to reach me, or send me anything I'll hopefully have access to email, but who knows how alert I'll be . . . Please don't ask too many questions about what the logistics look like, or where and when I'll be where and when—we just don't know that right now and will not for a little while. FOR INSTANCE:

Good message: "Wish Max well! No need to reply!"

Bad message: "When is Max next going to the bathroom, and in what city—I'd like to bring my schnauzer to visit him; he's a good luck healing massage schnauzer from Ireland. Is Max going to die? How often will Max die? Can he attend my event in four months?"

I love all of you very much, and am extremely grateful for your support.

The part about the "good luck healing massage schnauzer" made me smile. Max fancied himself a comedian and was always trying to make everyone laugh, even now, but once I was done reading, I thought about what this all meant—about the fact that he'd had multiple relapses since his first diagnosis at sixteen, and that in spite of all the treatments, the cancer continued to spread. The fucking cancer. The water in the tub felt like it was weighing down my limbs. I slipped beneath the surface again; this time, I closed my eyes and screamed.

Perhaps the greatest test of love is the way we act in times of need. It is the moment of accountability that all relationships seem to arc toward. I've prided myself on being a good friend in tough times—on being capable of sitting with hard things and going above what is required to be there for someone as they near the knife's edge. Over the last few years, I've sent care packages, bouquets, and musical telegrams. I've helped check items off bucket lists, been a third wheel on a Make-A-Wish adventure, organized meal deliveries, set up fundraisers, and sat vigil in hospice.

But as I thought about Max, it felt as if my well for such gestures had run dry. I didn't even have it in me to respond. As I got out of the tub and went to bed, I told myself, *Tomorrow.*

Now "tomorrow" is here and I still haven't reached out.

I press down on the accelerator, the pedal quivering beneath my foot. *No. No. No,* I think as I drive along a frozen stretch of highway. *I cannot go through this again.* There is no greater cruelty than being met with silence from a friend who you thought would be one of the first to say, *I'm here, I love you, what can I do?* I know this firsthand. But right now my impulse is self-preservation. It's to withdraw, to hedge against the pain of losing him, too. The thought of more heartbreak makes me want to cut myself off from the world. I wish to never get close to another person again.

I take Highway 141 toward Avon, Montana. It's the type of rural ranching community where the cattle far outnumber the human inhabitants. I'm on my way to visit Salsa, the ranch cook who sent me a care package when I was in the hospital, promising to feed me in abundance if I ever found myself in these parts. She'd given me detailed, albeit cryptic, directions for how to find her family's ranch. When I asked her for an address or coordinates, suggesting that it might be easier to simply plug this information into my GPS, Salsa's response had been: *Go with God on that one.*

I travel three miles down a dirt road. When I spot the small shed Salsa described—it's wood with a painting of a blue-and-gold quilt on the side—I take an immediate right, my tires skidding slightly on ice. I rumble over a cattle guard and onto another dirt road, winding toward the green ranch house up the hill. As I approach, Salsa runs outside. With her round, rosy cheeks, and blond hair poking out from beneath a winter hat, she looks like she could be cast in the local Christmas pageant as Mrs. Claus. Her smile splits wide as I get out of the car, and she jumps up and down in her boots and anorak, woo-hooing with infectious enthusiasm. "Welcome to our big-ass, beautiful state! We've all been peeing our pants a little at the thought of you coming," she says, squashing me into her bosom.

Salsa tells me she's been preparing for my visit for days and has made enough food to feed a fleet of cowboys—trays of lasagna, sheets of her famous chocolate chip cookies baked to gooey perfection, and heaps of caramelized popcorn balls for late-night snacking. She swept the little bunkhouse on the ranch where I will stay, made up the bed with a hand-sewn quilt, and lit a fire in the woodstove so that it would be toasty by the time I arrived. As if this wasn't enough, she has gotten me a "real Montana hat"—a Davy Crockett–style coonskin cap with a long black-and-brown ringed tail hanging off the back.

This is the type of person Salsa is: She loves hard and holds nothing back. I first got a glimpse of her generous spirit two years earlier when we met briefly at what we called "cancer camp"—a free weeklong outdoor adventure program put on by a nonprofit called First Descents for young adults with cancer.

Salsa was there in the capacity of "camp mom," as she invited everyone to call her. She had volunteered to cook three meals a day and to make sure all of us were well taken care of for the week. She had a nurturing presence and a saucy sense of humor that drew me to her right away. Whenever I was too tired to partake in camp activities, I sought refuge in the kitchen, where she plied me with brownies, still hot from the oven, and made me snort with laughter as she ranked the counselors—all of them strapping young outdoorsmen—in order of hunkiness. She also took swigs from a bottle of illicit whiskey that she hid from "camp authorities" inside a zippered purse decorated with Bible verses, which made me like her even more.

I'd loved every minute of my time at cancer camp. The counselors taught us to kayak and we spent hours drifting down the river each day, the thought of doctors' appointments and chemo receding with every paddle stroke. I stopped fixating on how my body had failed me, or worrying about the ways in which it struggled to keep up now, and focused instead on the smaller victories—mustering the guts to jump off a cliff into the river, learning to do a "sweep roll" in my kayak, and navigating a set of rapids without flipping over. By the end of the week, I was bruised and sore, but I felt proud of my body for the first time since my diagnosis.

I returned home brimming with resolutions to be someone "out living it," as the camp's motto proclaimed. I resolved to leave the city on weekends for hikes and I proposed to Will that we go on a camping trip in the Adirondacks. But soon after I returned, I was hospitalized with a bronchial infection and hooked up to an oxygen tank for days. Somehow Salsa found out I was in the hospital, and she immediately overnighted me a package containing a beautiful glass bluebird to hang in the window of my room and a card inviting me to visit her in Montana once I was well enough. *You could come to my daughter's ranch, meet some real cowboys and ride the range on horseback,* she wrote. Lying there, in my hospital bed, I'd tried to picture the ranch in my mind's eye. I saw mountains, white massifs jutting up mightily from the earth. I imagined myself on horseback galloping through the woods. The beeping of my monitor jerked me back to reality. The oxygen tank that hissed air through a tube in my nostrils had become unhooked. Montana was thousands of miles away.

Within minutes of arriving, Oscar starts chasing the chickens. Around and around the barn they go. Oscar's running as fast as he can, ears flapping in the wind, but he has trouble keeping up on his stumpy legs. He's gunning after one chicken in particular, a portly russet hen who squawks as she flees from him, seemingly less frightened than irritated by his pursuit.

"I'm sorry," I say to Salsa. "I don't think he's ever seen a chicken before."

"Honey, I'm not worried," Salsa says. "No offense, but from the looks of your pup, I doubt he'd be able to catch much of anything." It doesn't help Oscar's image that he's dressed in a plaid red-and-black winter coat.

Salsa's daughter Erin joins us outside, and the three of us look on at the spectacle, laughing. Even the ranch dogs—tough herding mutts with missing front teeth from getting kicked one too many times by cattle—seem to smile. But as the minutes pass, Oscar gains speed, his tiny paws whirring through the air, his brown eyes glossing over with determination as he inches closer to the hen. And then it happens: Oscar flies forward in a fantastic lunge and catches the hen by her tail feathers.

"Oh shit, no no nononooo," I shout, breaking into a sprint. I grab Oscar by the collar and clip his leash back on, and as I do, Erin inspects the hen, which is thankfully unharmed. "Good thing my husband isn't here," she says. "A rancher'll shoot a dog for going after a chicken."

Whereas Salsa is plump and fair, Erin has dark, luminous eyes, long chestnut hair, and the wiry, muscular build of a woman who never stops moving. When Erin's not running the household, looking after the kids, sewing quilts on commission, and leading Bible study, she's helping her husband wrangle the cattle. The ranch, she tells me, has been in her husband's family for five generations.

Despite the scuffle with the chicken, Erin and I take a liking to each other right away. We head up to the green ranch house on the hill. Inside, we all take off our boots and line them up against the wall beside a wood-burning stove. "Let me give you a tour," she says, hooking her arm through mine. I follow her around the house, and she points out the bedrooms and the mountain views, then takes me into the cellar, where the shelves are filled with an impressive stockpile of canned goods, provisions, and whiskey—or as they call it, "hooch." "We hunt, gather, and grow pretty much everything we need right here from our land," Erin says proudly.

We head back upstairs to the kitchen, and I do what I can to make myself helpful as she and Salsa prepare an omelet soufflé and thick slabs of bacon. Summoned by the warm smells, Erin's four kids appear in the kitchen doorway and gawk at me with curiosity. They attend a three-room schoolhouse down the road where the other students are also the sons and daughters of ranchers. They wear work boots to class, attend 4-H as an extracurricular, and make jokes about cow farts, Salsa says, ruffling the hair of the youngest boy, Finn.

When the kids are out of earshot, Erin tells me she's also been sick. "Cervical cancer," she whispers. It never ceases to surprise me just how many people I encounter who are living with some private struggle. The greater the distance I travel and the more people I encounter, the more convinced I've become that these human experiences bridge differences that might otherwise feel insurmountable.

As I help set the table, Erin's husband, William, arrives. He's dressed in his ranching clothes—a wool cap, silk neckerchief, snug-fitting Carhartt jacket, blue jeans, and leather boots. He has an impressive beard, so long and fluffy that it looks like it could be a nesting place for birds. He tips his cap cordially at me and takes a seat at the head of the big wooden table.

"Let's say grace," William begins. My body stiffens when everyone reaches out to hold hands. I've never said grace in my life but it seems rude not to partake, so I bow my head and close my eyes. He then leads us in prayer, short and sweet: "Thank you, Lord, for this day and this food, and bless it to the nourishment of our bodies. Amen."

·   ·   ·

Each week, the ranchers' wives gather for an aerobics class in town, which consists of the three-room schoolhouse, a post office, and a small gymnasium. Erin invites me to come, and Salsa tags along. The gym is brightly lit with polished wood floors that squeak beneath our sneakers. About a dozen women, spanning several decades, stretch in windbreakers and sweat suits. They stare at me as I am introduced; I get the sense they don't get many outsiders here. I imagine that my foreign name doesn't help much either. But when Erin begins to tell the women about my road trip, they listen with curiosity, and at the mention of the word "leukemia," their faces visibly soften.

"Welcome," one of the women says. "I'm a survivor, too."

"We're glad to have you join us," another tells me.

"Have you met William's brother?" a third jumps in. "He's single. And real handsome."

"Wait! If you marry William's brother, we'd be sisters!" Erin exclaims.

"About time we find you a real cowboy, not some Yankee city slicker," Salsa adds playfully.

When it comes to working out, the ranchers' wives do not mess around. Over the course of the next hour, we move around the length of the gym where, at each station in an exercise circuit, we endure some new kind of abuse. We do jumping jacks until our legs tremble, squats until our glutes burn, and burpees until we are ready to collapse. But much to my surprise and satisfaction, I'm able to keep up.

Afterward, I go to wash up and in the bathroom mirror, I am met with a reflection I vaguely recall. My complexion used to have the moonlight pallor of silver birch, but now my cheeks are flushed and my eyes shine. Endorphins flow through my body like electricity, and I feel strong, energized. I smooth the jagged tips of my hair, now long enough that I can just about tuck it behind my ears— *very nineties Leonardo DiCaprio,* I think to myself. I am nothing like the girl who left home nearly fifty days ago. I am a sojourner, an adventurer, a road warrior, crushing the big miles, even if I still go to sleep shattered with exhaustion at the end of each day.

Later that evening, we all gather in the bunkhouse for dinner. William's brother shows up, every bit as handsome as everyone says, and he keeps stealing shy glances at me from across the room. Outside, the temperature has dropped to well below freezing, and Salsa tells me it isn't uncommon for the temperature to get as low as negative thirty at night. They heat their house with a woodstove, using logs that William chopped himself. Even with a fire crackling and long johns underneath my jeans it's the kind of cold that makes me wonder if I will ever be warm again. They pass out mugs of hooch, and the whiskey warms our insides a little more with each sip. Once the brothers have a good enough buzz going, their diffidence melts away and they join in the conversation.

"So, what do you have for protection?" William asks, turning to me.

"What do you mean? Like, birth control?" I ask.

Salsa guffaws, spitting her beer.

"No," William clarifies, frowning a bit. "Like a gun. For safety."

"Oh, no, nothing like that. I've never touched a gun in my life. I'd sooner end up accidentally shooting myself in the foot than brandishing it in self-defense. Nope, it's just me and little man," I say, giving Oscar a pat.

"Aren't you afraid?" William's brother asks. They seem disturbed by the thought that I've traveled all these miles without even a pocketknife. A woman with a small, neutered lapdog for protection shouldn't travel unarmed, they insist. William offers to give me one of his guns to take with me on the road. I decline, but only after we strike a compromise: I won't leave the ranch until I've learned how to shoot a tin can from at least twenty feet away—a challenge that will take me the better part of the next afternoon.

For our dinner, we feast on elk sausage, then bowls of Erin's beef stew. They tell me that the elk was one William had hunted, and they'd raised the cow themselves. "I don't like to be dependent on anything or anybody," William says. He spends a few moments expounding on his suspicions of government, public schools, even doctors. "We have everything we need to survive and to protect ourselves right here."

As the night goes on, William's brother moves to the couch and sits next to me. He has a ginger beard and blue eyes, and wears a flannel shirt. He speaks sparingly, but even so, I get the sense that he might like me. I can feel his eyes on me as I talk, and when I catch his gaze, we both blush. These days, I'm always surprised when men pay me a certain type of attention. While in treatment, I'd felt scrubbed of my sexuality altogether. No one catcalled as my mother rolled me down the street in a wheelchair. No one's eyes roved over my skeletal silhouette, unless it was to do a double take at the catheter tubes poking out from above my neckline. If anything, people averted their eyes. Now, whenever men flirt with me, I don't feel compelled to set a boundary or mention that I'm in a relationship. I relish the attention, even crave it.

Our knees brush and, for a moment, I allow myself an absurd fantasy about a life with William's brother on the ranch. Stability for me has always been in someone's arms, no matter how fleeting the time there. Whenever I am feeling lost or stuck, it's been my pattern to end whatever relationship I am in and immediately find my compass in a new man. This has always been a convenient way to avoid figuring out what I want for myself or working on the problems at hand. It's easier to fixate on a new love interest than to face what's really at stake. But I know what a self-deceptive trick this is, so I stand up, say good night to my cowboy suitor, and head to bed.

The next afternoon, we all troop to an empty clearing on the out-skirts of the woods, where William lines up six cans on a fallen log. I'm wearing my new coonskin cap and can't help feeling a bit ridiculous as William teaches me how to load bullets and fire. I start off with a pistol—otherwise known as a "lady gun," they tell me—for practice. After a couple shots, William deems me ready to graduate to a long rifle. "The kick'll knock your teeth out if you're not careful," he says. "Hold it against your shoulder." He adjusts my posture.

It's an old .22, the same rifle that William used to teach his kids how to shoot gophers before they moved on to hunting the elk that throng the woods. When I pull the trigger, my shoulder jerks back from the blast, my nostrils filling with the acrid scent of gunpow-der. After more than a dozen tries, I finally manage to hit one of the tin cans, and Erin and Salsa whoop loudly, their cheers echoing through the woods.

We head back toward the house, and I pack my things and load up the car. Salsa and her family gather around to say goodbye and give me more homemade cookies than I can possibly eat. "So, we've been talking," William says to me. "We've been talking, and we decided you can be on our list."

"Oh yeah?" I reply. "What list is that?"

"Our list of non–family members allowed to join us on the ranch in End Times," William says, appearing serious.

"Oh, wow, thank you," I say. My mind flickers back to their cel-lar, filled with enough canned provisions, emergency supplies, water canisters, and hooch to last a literal lifetime. Their suspi-cion of mainstream life, stash of guns, and insistence that they can hunt, gather, and grow everything they need on their own land all make sense to me now. Salsa and her family are survivalists. When I ask them about it, they explain that it's less of a lifestyle choice than a simple fact of life in this part of Montana. But when the world as we know it implodes, they will be prepared.

"Everyone on the list has to contribute in some way," Salsa butts in. "You have pretty much no practical skills—you don't know anything about cattle or ranching, and you can't shoot a gun for shit." She laughs, poking me with her elbow. "But maybe you can be our scribe."

There is something in this gesture, the idea that I am welcome here in spite of our differences, that moves me. The instinct to be self-sufficient, to cut yourself off from the world, to prepare for the worst—well, those are things I can relate to on some level. It's what I've been doing with Jon and now with Max, guarding my heart against more loss. But for this family, the idea of disaster breeds closeness and generosity. In the fear of death, they have found a source not of alienation, but of intimacy.

As I leave the ranch, my phone pings. It's a message from a number I don't recognize. The text says: *Come back to visit—your Montana husband (William's brother).* I expected to feel burned-out, maybe even homesick, by the time I completed the last leg of my journey west. Instead, as I head toward Seattle, I feel none of those things, only spellbound by this country's wild landscapes and the vibrant characters who've so generously welcomed me into their lives. I wonder if this sense of awe is what it means to feel alive again.

33

"DOING A BROOKE"

AS A YOUNG woman traveling alone, I've gotten a lot of unsolicited advice from strangers. Everywhere I go—eating at a roadside diner, waiting in line for the washroom at a campground, pumping gas at a truck stop—I meet people with wisdom they'd like to impart.

Some of the advice has been less than helpful. Before my departure, one wealthy acquaintance mentioned that it might be safer if I hired "a chauffeur" for my road trip. ("Oh! Great suggestion," I replied politely.) Other bits of advice have been more practical. I stayed for a night on the Oregon coast with a fisherman named Brent who gave me solid driving tips. "When your windshield starts to fog up, press the car dehumidifier thingy," he said. "Otherwise, you won't be able to see and you'll be screwed." Another host, Wendy—a legendary Portland actress, comedian, and self-described "senior citizen battling food addiction and 'CJPD: Chronic Jewish Personality Disorder'"—offered sound instructions on how to get out of a funk: "1) Write a list of things you are grateful for 2) Get your head out of your ass and take a walk out-side 3) If you don't have an eating disorder, get some good fucking chocolate and a strong cup of coffee."

Then, there's the advice that has been so prescient it's uncanny, advice that shakes up my inner kaleidoscope, allowing things to settle in a different light. Take Isaac, a young man I met in Seattle; he'd just driven there from rural Alaska, with all of his worldly belongings packed into his trunk. We were staying in the same guesthouse, and he spent much of the weekend on the verge of tears, telling me about his wife who'd just left him. He was be-reft, but clearheaded. "Forgiveness is a refusal to armor your own heart—a refusal to live in a constricted heart," he said, seemingly as much to himself as to me. "Living with that openness means feeling pain. It's not pretty, but the alternative is feeling nothing at all."

Night falls swiftly, a pale slant of moonlight streaking the dirt driveway as I pull up to the wooden gates of a home in Humboldt County. This isn't one of my planned visits. When I mentioned to Brent, the fisherman, that I was looking for a place to stay in Northern California, he gave my number to his son-in-law, who in turn gave it to a friend of his named Rich, who called me up earlier this morning, offering to let me stay the night in a cabin on his property.

Rich welcomes me with a big, warm smile, the crow's-feet around his gray eyes crinkling. His wife, Joey, is at choir practice so it's just the two of us for dinner. "I hope you don't mind vegan food," he says as I follow him inside.

As he bustles around the kitchen, Rich tells me he's a retired psychologist who now, in his free time, makes sculptures. The house contains several of his creations, twisting statuettes hand-carved from wood. I'm taken by one in particular. It's bizarrely beautiful, carnal and ethereal—a figure writhing, unfolding, in the middle of a metamorphosis. Rich tells me he made it out of the base of a massive maple tree. He calls it *Koschey's Egg*, and explains how in Slavic folklore, Koschey was a sorcerer who hid his soul inside nested objects, like a duck's egg buried under the roots of a mighty tree, so as to remain immortal. He says he draws a lot from his experience as a psychologist: "I'm interested in how people who are broken by life events are pushed to enter a place where the answers lie beyond our rational and emotional capacities."

I nod as he says this. His words certainly resonate.

We sit in the living room, next to a large adobe fireplace. Over our meal of roasted squash, kale salad, and kalamata olives, Rich regales me with tales of traveling around Europe in a van with his wife and sons in the mid-eighties. He has a theory: When we travel, we actually take three trips. There's the first trip of preparation and anticipation, packing and daydreaming. There's the trip you're actually on. And then, there's the trip you remember. "The key is to try to keep all three as separate as possible," he says. "The key is to be present wherever you are right now."

This advice, more than any, stays with me.

Early the next morning, I rise and begin driving down the California coast with Rich's theory still ringing in my ears—trying to stay anchored in *this road trip*, without letting my thoughts time-travel. Reaching the West Coast signals a turning point. I've gone as far as I can without driving into the ocean. It's hard not to fret about what comes next. It's hard not to think about returning to New York City, and what will happen then. I thought I'd have more answers by now. What I have instead are more questions.

When I see a trail marker for the Redwood National and State Parks to the side of the road, I pull over to let Oscar out. *So what's the big deal with these redwoods, anyway?* I wonder, glancing at the informational placard at the trailhead as I wait for Oscar to finish peeing. Curious, I decide to take a little hike.

The ocean fog from the Pacific, low and rolling, plumes through the forest. Oscar and I pad along a three-mile path, the sound of our footsteps absorbed by moss. As the path wends deeper, the trees around us grow taller, their leaves knitting together overhead in a thick canopy. I pause in front of an exceptionally large redwood that bears the black, burnt bark of fire scars and touch my fingertips to its trunk. The redwoods are the last remaining species of a genus that dates back to as early as the Jurassic period. They've managed not only to survive and to adapt, but to make space for others, sprouting and supporting new life, new growth— the hanging gardens of ferns dripping from their branches, the wisps of chartreuse lichen furring their bark, the huckleberry bushes sipping strength from their soil.

When we reach the end of the trail, Oscar stops to lap from a pool of water and I take a seat on a rock to catch my breath. Dropping my head back, I peer up at the sky. Topping three hundred feet, the redwoods seem to be omniscient, clairvoyant giants arrowing toward the heavens, overlooking the land. *What do you see that I can't? Where do I go from here?* I want to ask them. As I listen to the high-up branches creak in the wind, my breathing slows and deepens. It strikes me that the redwoods have accomplished, without effort or ego, what I have struggled so hard to do. They make existence, as I conceive of it—time measured in hundred-day increments—seem laughably naïve and nearsighted. I feel so tiny and rootless in their midst. Right now, I am no redwood. I am a speck, a spore surfing the breeze, directionless and susceptible, blown any which way, without the faintest clue about where I'll land.

I unzip my backpack and take out my journal. *Lately, every new place I visit, I find myself trying it on for fit,* I write. *Could I move to this town, this city, this region, this state? Could this be where I finally settle? Just last night, I spent an hour before bed looking at real estate listings in Humboldt County and dreaming about buying land, somewhere quiet and remote, some place I can call my own. In this fantasy, I live alone, with only my books and a couple of dogs to keep me company.*

Later that afternoon, I set up camp in a state park in Big Sur, pitching my tent on the edge of a meadow. The sun lowers, its light spreading across the ocean like a broken egg yolk. The air is warm enough that I don't have to zip the flap of my tent closed right away. I lie spread eagle on top of my sleeping bag, with my muddy boots poking out of the tent. Copying me, Oscar flops onto his back, all four paws in the air. I reach over to rub his belly and he gazes up at me with helpless love. Living on the road together 24/7 has turned us into an old couple who mirror each other's gestures without realizing it and know exactly what the other needs without having to inquire. It's hard to believe it's already been more than three years since I brought him home. "Congratulations, you're officially my longest, most successful adult relationship yet," I say, turning to face Oscar, who replies by licking my nose.

If only all relationships could be so uncomplicated, I think. I sigh as my thoughts turn to Jon. I've been too confused to know what to say to him. Other than the text messages we exchange—where he asks if I am safe and I say that I am, and I ask if he is well and he says that he is—we've barely spoken at all. Things between us feel tense and pulled taut, and it seems like any day now we might break apart.

If I could, I would revise the chronology of us. I would have waited to start dating him until I'd found my foothold among the living—or, at the very least, until I was no longer regularly crying over my ex. Maybe then things would have gone differently. But of course, this is the kind of time-travel thinking Rich was just warning me about. I can't alter what's already happened; I must decide what to do now. The truth is, I don't feel capable of loving Jon the way he deserves, much less deserving of the love he's shown me. It's not right of me to keep evading the phone calls of a man—a good man, a deeply kind and patient one, who has given me the space I need to figure my shit out—who is trusting that I will return to him once the road trip is over. I've been mired in transition for much of our relationship, and I'm starting to think it would be fairer to him if we end things for good.

Before I can chicken out, I pick up my phone and send Jon a text asking if we can talk. Staring at my screen, I watch the three little dots appear and disappear as he types something and deletes it. I can sense his apprehension through the screen as he formulates a reply. He finally settles on a message saying he's busy and asking if we can talk this weekend. I'm relieved. I think we both know what will come of this conversation, and neither of us is quite ready for it to happen tonight.

The next morning I make my way onto Highway 1, a 656-mile stretch of road that hugs the Pacific coastline from north of San Francisco to south of Los Angeles. The highway is narrow, an endless series of white-knuckle turns, climbing higher and higher, with only a pathetic metal guardrail to prevent cars from careening over the edge of the jagged cliffs and falling hundreds of feet down into the ocean. I'm muttering f-bombs, clenching the wheel with both hands, glancing in the rearview mirror as flashy sports cars and vintage convertibles line up behind me. As I pass strawberry fields and golden beaches filled with sunning seals, I've never felt so awestruck and terrified—or so carsick.

After four harrowing hours, I turn off Highway 1 and drive toward Ojai, a town nestled in the mountains about eighty miles northwest of Los Angeles. The land turns psychedelic against the twilight: a hilly moonscape awash in an eerie pink glow. I'm on my way to see Katherine, who wrote to me in the aftermath of her son

Brooke's suicide. Letter writing, she explained, was a practice inspired by him. He once wrote a letter to a scientist, telling him how much he appreciated and admired his research; the recipient was so impressed that he invited the young man to his office hours and ended up offering him a job. After that, sending letters of gratitude to strangers had come to be known in their family as "doing a Brooke." The idea was that if you wanted to connect with someone out in the world, someone far removed from your own life, someone who maybe even seemed unknowable, you didn't let the distance stop you—you said what the hell, and you wrote. Katherine had reached out to me in that spirit, thanking me for my column: *The power of story is to heal and to sustain,* she wrote. *And if we are brave enough to tell our own story, we realize we're not alone, again and again.*

Through a cloud of red dust, I pull up to a small white house that sits at the base of a mountain. Katherine, a high school English and French teacher, opens the screen door, all *bienvenues*. Her border collie, Atticus, shuffles over to the car, thumping his tail in welcome. Katherine looks dignified in a crisp white oxford tucked into jeans, a black flat-brimmed cowboy hat, and matching black cowboy boots with spurs. Her thick dark hair, streaked with gray, is so long it skims her waist.

When she proposes a quiet night in, just the two of us and our dogs, and a dinner of seared tuna steaks, I nod gratefully. We take our plates and wineglasses to the back porch. Looking out onto the darkening valley, we dive deep without any warm-up chatter, and as we speak, I feel like I've known her my whole life. I recognize myself in her posture, in the grief that flashes across her eyes in moments. I notice the words she chooses and the ones she omits. The connection between us is instant, the trust implicit.

When Katherine asks how I've been, I tell her the unvarnished truth: I've been driving with the ghost of my ex riding shotgun, and despite my best efforts to be present I feel chased by my past. I tell her about Melissa and the others I've lost; about Max, who is recuperating from surgery at his family's home in Los Angeles, and how I've been too much of a coward to call. I tell her about my relationship with Jon and how I've decided to tell him it's over the next time we talk.

Katherine doesn't flinch. She doesn't avert her eyes. She doesn't try to placate me with platitudes or direct me with advice. She listens with her whole body, leaning forward in her seat, nodding ever so slightly as I speak. When I finish, she tells me she relates to all of it, and that she's so glad the universe saw fit for our paths to cross. "Grief isn't meant to be silenced," she says, "to live in the body and be carried alone."

We stand up and take our empty plates and glasses back inside the kitchen, then move into the living room, with its floor-to-ceiling shelves overflowing with books. On the coffee table there is a mandolin that Katherine tells me she's learning to play. I pause at the mantel, which is cluttered with framed photographs of her children—three girls and one boy. That must be Brooke, his handsome, intelligent face illuminated by votive candles.

The next afternoon I'm standing with Katherine in the stables near her house, where she has just given me a refresher course on how to ride a horse. She's a seasoned equestrian who goes on weeklong pack trips in the Sierra Nevada with her students and her beloved gelding, Blue, and she makes it look so easy as she mounts. I haven't been on horseback since I was a teenager and the pair of old cowboy boots I've borrowed from her are a size too big. I slip a little as I place my foot in the stirrup and attempt to hop up, nearly catapulting over the horse. But once I'm settled in the saddle, muscle memory takes over, and I quickly fall back into the posting rhythm as we trot through an orange grove, past her house, and onto a long winding trail that takes us up into the mountains.

Katherine tells me that Brooke loved to come out here to think. We approach an enormous sandstone boulder—"his favorite," she says—then dismounts her horse, walks over to the rock, and places her palm against a plaque engraved with Brooke's name.

"What was he like?" I ask.

"Oh, you two would have been such great friends," she says. "He was an extraordinary soul—a linguist-science-oriented-outdoorsman-climber-dude, and so joyful and wicked smart." She tells me about how he spoke fluent Mandarin and was interested in everything, from baking bread to organic chemistry. After graduating from college, Brooke moved to Vermont, where he worked as an arborist and volunteer firefighter. But Brooke had secretly struggled with depression since his freshman year of college, and in Vermont, he suffered a severe bout followed by his first manic episode. It was a terrifying descent into madness that landed him in a psychiatric hospital for weeks, and though Brooke tried to contain what he called his "demonic condition," he lost hope that he would ever be in control—at least not in a way that he could trust and depend on, in a way that those who loved him could trust and depend on. Bipolar disorder expresses itself differently in each organism it takes hold of, Katherine tells me. Like any disease, some cases are more virulent than others, some organisms more vulnerable. On a cold morning in November 2009, Brooke took his own life. He was twenty-six years old.

Gazing at the boulder, Katherine's face is radiant with grief. "He had an extraordinarily powerful mind that was equally powerful in illness," she says, as tears streak her cheeks.

"We don't have to talk about it if it's too painful," I say.

"Actually, it's healing for me to talk about Brooke and I appreciate you asking about him. People treat suicide as a shameful secret—leave the true cause of death unmentioned in the obituary, just erase it from the family narrative. But talking about the ones we've lost keeps them alive."

Katherine tells me Brooke wrote a letter before he died. When she reads it to me later, I'm floored: It is a rescue rope of compassion and love in which he attempts to answer the inevitable question of why. His letter, which reads almost as a living document, one that will support his loved ones in different phases of their grief, is clear-eyed and comprehensive. Brooke says he knows they will ask if they could have done more, and he assures them they did everything they could. He knows they will suffer, but he hopes it won't be more than what he would have gone through had he stayed. He tells them that whatever happens, he has faith in their ability to continue on. He says he is sorry and that he loves them over and over, too many times to count. It is generous and loving and—mired even as Brooke was in his own pain—you can feel him reaching out to his family from across a great gulf. It's his final way of "doing a Brooke."

To lose a child to suicide is a devastating, unimaginable, impossible tragedy to live through, a loss I can't begin to fathom—but Katherine's story doesn't end there. As we trot up the trail, she tells me about how, just four months after Brooke's death, she was out riding when her horse fell and she broke her leg. Not long after that, she went in for her first routine colonoscopy and learned she had colon cancer. She says it was an out-of-body experience—one of those moments where you think, *This can't* possibly *be my life*—but somehow it also felt mystically coherent. "Grieving is an emotional experience as well as a physical one," she says. "The fact that my bones broke and the cancer occurred in my gut felt symbolically appropriate."

When I ask Katherine how she dealt with it—how she shouldered the weight of sorrow upon sorrow—she pauses, slowing her horse. "Being stuck on bed rest was an invitation to unplug from the daily rhythms of teaching and responsibility, and to actually *experience* my grief," Katherine says. She turns and gestures to a white pickup truck in the distance, parked off to one side of her house. Going home without Brooke after the memorial service was really hard, she tells me. When she traveled to Vermont to pick up his things, she decided to take his truck and to drive it back across the country. It was a way of bringing him home. Brooke's truck had a front license plate from his volunteer fire department, and at gas stations and roadside diners along the way, people would notice it and make grateful comments. When they did, she would find herself welling up—not with sadness but pride. There was also a sense of ritual in the drive—in its great distance and its slow pace. It offered her essential time to understand that the unthinkable had happened, and to begin to accept it as her new reality.

Katherine tells me that Brooke's death has changed her relationship to her own mortality. Her cancer has returned twice since her initial diagnosis and she recently underwent yet another surgery, this time a thoracotomy to remove a nodule from her lungs. It's easier now to grapple with the thought that cancer might be the end of her story. "If my child can pass from this physical plane, surely I can figure out how to do that, too." She tilts her head, then continues. "The death bit doesn't scare me. It's the suffering that's hard."

To keep going, Katherine reminds herself every day of all the ways her life has been enriched—blessed by Brooke and his life, by her daughters and her grandchildren, by Atticus and Blue, and finally by the presence of grief itself. "Ultimately, the events of the last few years have been a terrible lesson in being present—and not just being present in my own life, but being present in the lives of the people I love," she says. "Tomorrow may happen, tomorrow may not."

Later that night, once the horses have been returned to their stalls, the dogs walked, the dinner eaten, and the dishes washed, I retreat to the spare bedroom. Sprawled across the bed, I open my journal and begin to revisit all the ways I've tried to do the opposite of Katherine—to avoid actually experiencing pain. Numbing out on everything from morphine to marathons of *Grey's Anatomy*. Denying that it's there at all. Refusing to let people in. I see now that these tactics have not rid me of my sorrow, just transmuted it, delayed it. *What if I stopped thinking of pain as something that needs to be numbed, fixed, dodged, and protected against? What if I tried to honor its presence in my body, to welcome it into the present?*

I used to think healing meant ridding the body and the heart of anything that hurt. It meant putting your pain behind you, leaving it in the past. But I'm learning that's not how it works. Healing is figuring out how to coexist with the pain that will always live inside of you, without pretending it isn't there or allowing it to hijack your day. It is learning to confront ghosts and to carry what lingers. It is learning to embrace the people I love now instead of protecting against a future in which I am gutted by their loss. Katherine's experience and her insight sit with me. She went through something she thought she could never survive and yet here she is, surviving. "You have to shift from the gloom and doom and focus instead on what you love," she told me before bed. "That's all you can do in the face of these things. Love the people around you. Love the life you have. I can't think of a more powerful response to life's sorrows than loving."

I close my journal and do the two things I've been avoiding for too long. First, I write an email to Max. Then, I call Jon. He picks up on the first ring.

"How far are you from Los Angeles?" he asks me.

"About an hour. Maybe two. What's up?"

"I'm booking a plane ticket and I'll be there tomorrow. We should have this conversation in person."

The next morning I dress in my road uniform—a pair of battered boots, black Levi's, a white T-shirt, and a favorite leather jacket I've had since college. I share a last cup of coffee with Katherine, who gives me her old road almanac as a parting gift, and I stoop down to give Atticus a scratch behind the ears. "Thanks for everything," I say, as I get into the car. "You've helped me more than you'll ever know."

I drive to Los Angeles and when I arrive at the airport, Jon is waiting for me on the curb outside the passenger pickup area, wearing a cotton scarf I got him in India and looking as dapper as ever. He spots me in the queue of cars, and though we try to steel our faces into an appropriately somber expression, we both split into dopey grins. As he gets into the car, we hug tightly, forgetting, for a moment, why he's made this last-minute trip.

"I'm so happy you're here," I say.

"You are?" Jon asks, pulling away. From the stiffness in his voice I can tell he's been hurting, and I feel a rush of tenderness toward him. I can't imagine this was an easy trip for him to make given how hectic his schedule has been. But I'm also not surprised that he's traveled all the way across the country to have this conversation in person. Jon has always shown up for me in difficult moments, even long before we were a couple.

We have so much to tell each other that at first only silence will do. As we drive, I think about how, when Jon learned of my diagnosis, he came straight to the hospital to see me with his whole band in tow. Jon had brought a melodica. Ibanda had his tuba, Eddie his sax, and Joe the drummer carried a tambourine. Right there in the middle of the cancer ward, they began to play for me. As the sound of "When the Saints Go Marching In" filled the hallways, nurses and patients filtered out of their rooms. The patients who could walk, walked; those who couldn't were wheeled to their doorways by nurses or family members. Others listened from their beds. Every inch of the ward was filled with music. Timidly at first, and then with jubilation, patients, nurses, and hospital workers began to dance and clap. The ward was breathing a sigh of relief, its inhabitants rejoicing in a temporary time-out, surrendering to the music. Beneath my face mask, I couldn't stop beaming.

Remembering all this, I'm no longer certain of what I'm about to do. Over the last few weeks, whenever I considered actually ending things between us, something in me had resisted picking up the phone. Now that we are together I feel even less confident, but I try, as I did the last few nights with Katherine, to tell the unvarnished truth. "I know I've been distant," I say as we inch through traffic. "It's been a struggle to figure out how to be in this relationship when there's so much I need to sort through alone. The two feel at odds with each other. If I'm being honest, I've spent a lot of my trip wondering if it would be best for us to break up."

"I want to ask you something," Jon says.

"What?"

"Do you like me?"

"Yeah, of course," I say.

"Tell the truth. Do you like being with me?"

"I do. I love you," I admit.

"Then why does everything need to be so dang complicated?"

We are both quiet for a while. "Listen," Jon says more gently, "maybe it's okay to not have the answers right now. I want to be with you. Even if that means continuing to give you space. I'm good with that. But what I do need is for you to be open and honest as we figure this out. You gotta stop shutting me out."

Over the last few weeks, I've put so much pressure on myself to be either fully in or fully out. I've been so caught up in assessing the risks and armoring myself against them that it hasn't occurred to me that there is a third way: to let things grow and change and evolve, to uncover who we are and what we want along the way—to live in that middle terrain. As I slow toward a stoplight, I reach over and squeeze his hand.

"We cool?" Jon asks.

"We cool," I reply.

"Not so fast," he says. "C'mere." And I do.

We kiss until the traffic light turns green and the drivers behind us start honking. I'm not sure what it all means. You can't force clarity when there is none to be had yet. But for as long as I've known him, Jon has been teaching me that sometimes all you can do is show up. And when things are hard, to keep on showing up.

Before leaving Los Angeles, I make one last stop. Through smog and rush-hour traffic, I drive to Brentwood, an affluent neighborhood with gated villas and impeccably landscaped lawns tended by teams of gardeners. It's my first time visiting Max's family home, and when I knock, his mother, Ari, and her standard poodle appear at the door. As we make chitchat in an opulent foyer, a very pale Max descends the stairs. He looks terribly skinny, his cheeks scooped hollow, making his blue eyes, already magnified by his glasses, appear even larger. He says hi in a gravelly baritone, explaining his voice is hoarse from the tumors in his chest, and leads me to his bedroom, where we can talk in private. He sits on the edge of his bed and I sit across from him in the desk chair, swiveling back and forth anxiously until he reaches out to steady me.

I stare at the rug, chewing on my lip, afraid that if I meet his eye I will turn into a puddle. "I know I haven't been there for you," I say, my voice quavering. I tell him how many times in the last weeks I've wanted to pick up the phone and call. I tell him I know better—that I've been on the receiving end of that kind of silence before—and that I understand if he can't forgive me. "There's no excuse for how cowardly I've been. I'm so sorry."

Max doesn't let me off the hook. It's not his style. "I've noticed your distance," he says evenly. "I'm not angry. I guess I just want to understand. Does it make you uncomfortable to know I'm dying?"

"Uncomfortable? No," I answer. "It terrifies me." I tell Max I didn't know it was possible to have a friendship with so much depth and understanding, and odds are, I will never have that again. He's the only person I can call in the middle of the night when I'm feeling worried about an upcoming biopsy—or to whom I can extol the virtues of Magic Mouthwash, without having to explain. He was there at Melissa's memorial, there every day of my last hospitalization, there every evening that first week after Will moved out. "You know me well enough to show up at my door even when I say I want no visitors—*especially* when I say I want no visitors," I tell him. "You hold me accountable, even now. You are the funniest, smartest, weirdest person I know, and I can't bear the thought of losing you."

"I get it," Max says, reaching over and tugging me up. "I figured as much. I forgive you. But I do need you now." He hugs me hard, with every sinew and muscle in his body, the kind of hug that crushes your lungs in a good way. Max has always given the best hugs.

When we sit back down, I ask Max what's been happening with his health, and he tells me he has started a new drug that is supposed to be really mild on the side effects. "But we all know how that goes," he says. "This is the worst pain I've been in in my entire life, and there may only be two or three hours a day when I can function. But in those two or three hours, I am Max, and it is good to be Max."

Over the next few hours, our conversation is an uninterrupted stream. He asks me about all the different people I've met and the places I've seen. I ask him about how married life is going and we reminisce about his wedding a few months earlier. Like me and Jon, Max and his wife, Victoria, met as teenagers, at a summer program. They were close friends for nearly a decade before they became a couple. Though he was in the middle of chemo, Max knew from the early weeks of their relationship that he was going to ask Victoria to marry him on the anniversary of their first date. Max is a master of impermanence, and I remember being awed by the radical hope and optimism embedded within his decision to propose, despite his prognosis. When he asked me if I would be one of his groomsmen, I'd felt honored. The wedding was held in Topanga Canyon, at an inn surrounded by old sycamores, water-falls, and wildflowers. His mentor, the poet Louise Glück, had of-ficiated at the ceremony.

Max tells me he's been reading Louise's book *Averno,* and that it's a masterpiece—the kind of book that only the wisdom of de-cades can bring you, something that you must die many times to be able to create. "Every time I've had a significant trauma, my writing has grown, I've grown," he says. "I think I could have writ-ten a masterpiece if I lived to fifty. If I had more time." There's an edge to his voice, a hardness I've never heard before. "I am bitter," he concedes. "It's struck me recently how strange it is, being this young and knowing that I'm going to die. It's very, very lonely."

He pauses, looking sadder than I've ever seen him. He says his life has been rich and fast—the best family, the best friends, the best wife, and his first book of poems coming out in just a couple months. "It's been delightful to see it all flower so quickly," he says. "Nothing is missing. But I would much rather have had a slow burn."

Max's voice has grown hoarser still and he looks tired. "Right now, I want to roll a joint, watch an episode of *The Bachelorette,* and rave with you about how awful it is, but I should probably take a nap," he says.

As I stand up to leave, I tell Max I love him and promise to call every couple of days with updates from the road. "It's incredible to me that you can be alone with your thoughts in a car for so long, when you've gone through what you've gone through," he says. "People have been experimenting on you for years and years, and you have the balls to experiment on yourself—to push your-self to grow. Now, *that* is strength."

"Oh, Max," I say. I clutch my heart dramatically. "I don't know what I'd do without your support."

"You are such an inspiration," he says.

"God doesn't give you more than you can handle," I say.

"Every day is a gift," he says.

With that, he gives me a last, lung-crushing embrace before I step out the door.

As I leave California, I cross the Mojave Desert, passing flowering cacti and yucca trees under a vast black sky prickling with stars. I don't know what will come of my relationship with Jon or if I will ever see Max again, but I no longer want to protect my heart. You can't guarantee that people won't hurt or betray you—they will, be it a breakup or something as big and blinding as death. But evading heartbreak is how we miss our people, our purpose. I make a pact with myself and send it off into the desert: *May I be awake enough to notice when love appears and bold enough to pursue it without knowing where it will lead.*

34

HOMEGOING

UNDER HEAVY SNOWFALL, Oscar and I huddle inside the tent, sleeping chest-to-chest like conjoined twins. I wake up on the morning of Day 66 at a campground outside of the Grand Canyon. A sense of longing fills my body as I rise and fire up my stove with numb fingers, shivering as I make coffee. It follows me as I pack up my tent for the umpteenth time and load my gear back into the car. Over the next few days, it intensifies as I drive through the martian landscapes of the Southwest and celebrate my first Hanukkah at the home of a Twitter acquaintance in Tijeras, New Mexico. Wandering around Santa Fe's snowy streets alone—the storefronts strung with pine garlands, the sidewalks bustling with families doing their holiday shopping—leaves me feeling a little blue.

Eventually, it dawns on me that, for the first time since hitting the road, I want to go home. I want to go home. *I want to go home*—an aching that becomes a kind of chant in my head as I drive. But home where? Without a job, a family of my own, or a

mortgage awaiting me, the concept feels tinny, weightless, as it
floats around in my head. I need to be in New York City around
Day 100 to return the car to my friend and see my medical team—
but beyond that nothing is certain. I feel a heightened need to use
these final miles wisely, to find answers among the people I meet
and the places I go.

Down into Texas I go, driving through lonely border patrol checkpoints and past puffs of sagebrush until I reach Marfa, a dusty,
one-stoplight town in the middle of the Chihuahuan Desert, made
famous in the last few decades as a destination for lovers of art
and, more recently, Instagram. Marfa is meant to be a pit stop, but
I am intrigued by this bizarre place and its residents, a mix of
ranchers and writers and painters, and I end up staying for a bit.
Over the next three days, I befriend all kinds of characters—
a Texan heiress who offers to let me stay in the spare bedroom of
her bungalow, a troop of high school drama club students whose
play I go to one night, and two combat-boot-wearing antique dealers I meet during a museum tour who invite me back to their trailer
for a lethal mescal cocktail. As a woman traveling alone, I feel like
what Gloria Steinem described as a "celestial bartender": Strangers welcome me into their homes, share secrets with me that they
wouldn't disclose to a therapist, invite me to partake in their family traditions, and send me off with homemade pies.

On my last morning in Marfa, outside the public library, I meet
a couple around my age who pique my curiosity. "We call her Sunshine," they tell me, introducing their 1976 Volkswagen camper van
before they introduce themselves. Despite being nearly half a cen-
tury old, Sunshine looks as youthful and free-spirited as her owners. She's tangerine orange with windows adorned with curtains
sewn from a groovy flower fabric and a dashboard decorated with
feathers. She has two beds, hidden compartments for storage, and
a makeshift kitchen.

"Are you brewing kombucha?" I ask, pointing to a giant jug of fizzy amber liquid wedged between the front seats.

"I can teach you how. It's so easy and so good for you," says the young woman, who calls herself Kit. With intense blue eyes and wildflowers woven through her blond curls, she has an elfin charm. Her boyfriend, JR, who is tinkering with Sunshine's engine, has a ponytail and the broad shoulders of a linebacker. The two of them are deeply tan and turn-and-stare gorgeous. They tell me they've spent the last three years living out of the van.

I am instantly smitten with Sunshine and her inhabitants. I want to know everything about their lives. Where they've traveled. The things they've seen and the people they've met. What they do to make a living. How in the world they came to call this orange bus home.

"It was love at first gear," Kit and JR tell me. The van had been sitting for some months in a parking lot across the street from Appalachian State University in the North Carolina mountains where Kit was a student. After graduation, the couple, who had been dating since high school, bought the van for five thousand dollars, moved into a cramped studio apartment in Venice Beach, and got jobs—she as a waitress in a wine bar and he as a videographer for a surfing website. Suffocated by city life and unfulfilled by the long hours they spent working, they made an impulsive decision: They quit their jobs, gave up their apartment, and decided to try living on the road. Sunshine became not merely a traveling abode but a lifestyle, an ideology. Freed from the tyranny of nine-to-five, they started exploring the most remote corners of the country.

"We travel with the agricultural seasons," JR tells me when I ask how they can afford to keep their gas tank full. "We live on very little and whenever we need cash, we work as farmhands and migrant laborers for a month or two. Fruit harvesting, dairy farming, haying horses, digging ditches—you name it, we done it."

Instead of paying rent, Kit and JR set up camp in national parks and forests, redwood groves and deserts. They bathe in rivers and hot springs, cook every meal from scratch, and eat foods foraged from the earth. When they're not milking goats, harvesting peaches, or scaling mountains, they spend their days working on various creative projects. JR takes photographs and keeps his hands busy with woodworking. Given Sunshine's age, he's also become something of an amateur mechanic. Kit spends her days cooking, bird-watching, and studying metaphysics. She loves to write and to draw cartoons, and the two of them collaborate on little zines about their adventures.

I'm taken by the fact that JR and Kit have figured out how to make this transience a permanent way of life. Against the conventional benchmarks of success and societal expectations, they seem to have found a purpose in the endless promise of the open road. They strike me as proof that home doesn't need to be a place or a profession, that I might find it wherever I go.

JR slices up a loaf of farm bread, a block of cheddar, and some apples on a wooden cutting board while Kit refills our jars of kombucha. As we sit down for a snack in the back of Sunshine, we are joined by a smiling surfer with hair like straw named Mikey, who is traveling with them for the week. "We're headed to Big Bend National Park," they say as we eat. "Why don't you come with us and we can join camps for a night?"

I do a quick mental calculation. I've already spent longer in Marfa than planned. I'm supposed to be driving to Austin today. Big Bend is out of the way, a hundred miles south, and it will mean spending an intimidating number of hours behind the wheel over the next few days.

"Hell yes," I say.

We chug along all day in a caravan of two, with Sunshine at the front and my mud-splattered Subaru close behind. My new friends don't use GPS, and on account of Sunshine only going a maximum of fifty-five miles per hour, we avoid the highway. Instead, we stick to the small country roads that squiggle out into nowhere, leading to territories that feel untouched by civilization. As travelers, they are remarkably inefficient and whenever something catches their curiosity, they pull over to explore. If they like their surroundings, they'll stay for a while, entire days, sometimes weeks.

After a few hours, the Rio Grande appears, the winding emerald-hued ribbon that separates Texas from Mexico. We turn off the main road and bounce along a dirt path, grinding to a stop on a promontory overlooking the river valley. Cracked copper earth, unending blue sky, a jagged ravine that drops down to a sea of rippling gold grass—all of it feels like it belongs to us this afternoon as we scramble down rocks and hike through the heat until we reach the water's edge. Other than a couple of roadrunners and a little family of javelinas snuffling through the brush, it's been hours since we've seen another soul. My new friends ditch their clothes and jump into the water. I hesitate for a moment, then follow suit; it's too hot out here to be self-conscious about unsightly scars and unwieldy curves. As I wade in, the river is cool and viscous, its color and consistency turning into that of chocolate milk as the four of us shriek and splash around, kicking up silt. Even Oscar, who has never been much of a swimmer until now, barrels in snoutfirst.

As the sun descends, we drive a little farther, continuing offroad until we reach a secluded clearing at the base of a mountain with striated red cliff faces. While JR and Mikey are out gathering wood for a fire, I help Kit prepare dinner over their two-burner Coleman stove. Digging through one of the storage compartments, she pulls out a dusty bottle of wine they've been saving for a special occasion. Dusk falls like soot over our little camp as we gather for dinner, crammed together on the backseats with Oscar tuckered out at our feet. With the van's side doors flung open onto a crackling fire, we balance bowls on our knees, dunking chunks of bread into a savory stew, discussing everything from the opti-

mal frequency of washing one's hair to idle theory—their philoso-
phy that our lives should be less busy, more filled with leisure, with
days just like this.

Around midnight, I say good night to my new pals. Sleepy and
sun-whipped, I trip through the darkness toward my car. I'm too
tired to set up my tent so I haul all of my gear into the front seats
and fold the back ones down flat. In the empty cargo space, I layer
blankets and a sleeping bag over a foam camping mat. I'm pleased
to discover that my improvised bed is actually quite comfortable
and that there's just enough room for me to stretch out my legs.
With all of the windows rolled down and the hatchback popped
open, a warm breeze washes over me. All is quiet except for the
trembling of juniper trees and the occasional yips and howls of
coyotes in the distance. The night sky is powdered with more stars
than I've ever seen in my life.

Gazing up at the Milky Way, I remember when all I wanted is
what I have in this moment. Sitting on the kitchen floor of my old
apartment, sicker than I'd ever felt, my heart fractured into ten
thousand tiny pieces, I needed to believe that there was a truer,
more expansive and fulfilling version of my life out there. I had no
interest in existing as a martyr, forever defined by the worst things
that had happened to me. I needed to believe that when your life
has become a cage, you can loosen the bars and reclaim your freedom. I told myself again and again, until I believed my own words:
It is possible for me to alter the course of my becoming.

I scoot around in my sleeping bag with my toes pointing toward
the steering wheel and my head resting on the back bumper so that
I have an unobstructed view of the Big Dipper blinking down at
me. Within seconds, I spot a shooting star. Then another. Soon, I
see so many that I lose count. As I watch the sky sizzle and spark,
a warm, euphoric sensation seeps through my bones that can only
be described as joy. I am alive and as well as I could ever hope to

be. I have been entrusted with a life that I am making into my own. Tonight, this feeling is the closest I've felt to being at home within myself.

But as soon as I close my eyes, I lose sight of the shooting stars and my vision turns inward. I'm back to replaying the same old scenes in my head. The last time Will and I saw each other. A claustrophobically hot summer night, a few weeks before I left on my road trip. I remember hoping that enough time had passed for us to reach some sort of peace agreement. The conversation had started off cordially enough, but a couple of hours later, we'd ended up on the sidewalk in front of a bar in the East Village hurling accusations. Before parting ways, we came to an agreement on one thing, and one thing only: It was best if we didn't speak to or see each other again.

My chest constricts tighter and tighter. I want to be released from what won't let me go. I want uncomplicated joy. But I see now that, without realizing it, I've been waiting for permission— from Melissa, from Will, from all the people who have disappeared from my life before a sense of closure could be reached. I want their blessings to fall in love again, to dream a new future, to move forward. I keep waiting for some kind of sign, or reassurance that it's okay to go entire days without thinking of them—that it's necessary to forget a little if I am going to live. No matter how many apologies, acts of contrition, or sacrifices I offer up, I'm realizing I need to accept that things may never feel fully resolved—with the living or the dead.

The next morning I eat breakfast with the van dwellers and we part ways, promising to keep in touch. In the days that follow, I pass ghost towns, forests of prickly pear cacti, and enormous roadside billboards that say things like WHERE BBQ LOVERS MEAT UP. I drive through Austin, then hike around a swimming hole where the water is so aquamarine-clean it looks chlorinated. On I go, east across Texas, following interminable highways until they all begin to melt together. It's early evening when I pull into the parking lot of the Best Western on Highway 59 in Livingston, a depressing stretch of fast-food restaurants and chain stores near the Louisiana border. The receptionist, a woman in a candy-cane sweater with pink acrylic nails, hands me a room key. "Enjoy your stay, sweetheart," she says.

I chose the Best Western because it is the cheapest hotel I could find and because it is a ten-minute drive from the prison. Tomorrow morning, I am scheduled to visit Lil' GQ, the inmate who was one of the first strangers to write to me. Typically, inmates are only allowed a two-hour visit each week, but I'd been granted what's called a "special visit," which consists of two four-hour visits spread over two days and is usually reserved for close friends and family. Now that I'm here, the idea of spending eight hours with Lil' GQ makes me gnaw my cuticles. Eight hours feels like a very long time to commit to talking to anyone, let alone a stranger, let alone a stranger who has spent the last fourteen years on death row.

In my room on the second floor of the Best Western, I read the first letter Lil' GQ ever sent to me, reliving the bewilderment I'd felt in my hospital bed as I tried to imagine him in a prison cell halfway across the country. During those long, maddening stays in the Bubble, I'd thought about him often. I wanted to know what he did to pass the time in solitary. I wanted to ask: How do you continue on when your life, as you know it, is over? How do you confront the ghosts of your past? How do you live in the present when what lies ahead is terrifyingly unknown?

My room overlooks the parking lot. I can see my car from the window, coated in a thick film of dust and so muddy that it looks like it's been in a fight. It's getting late and I still need to grab a couple of things from the trunk before bed. I pull on my boots, head outside, and as I'm walking across the parking lot, I notice a group of men standing by a couple of pickup trucks. Something about the men gives me pause, a tug in my gut that tells me to turn around and to go back inside. It's the same instinctual uneasiness I felt during my first week on the road, at the campground in Massachusetts, when I'd spotted my tarp-dragging neighbor, Jeff, and his dog emerging from the woods—except, of course, Jeff had turned out to be not only harmless but a pretty nice guy. With him in mind, and all the other times I've fretted for nothing and then felt silly, I ignore the warning bells in my head.

I'm rooting through the hatchback in search of a tube of toothpaste and some kibble for Oscar when I hear a wolf whistle, low and throaty, slicing through the dark. "Come on over here and talk to us for a minute," one of the men calls out. I ignore him and his friends. I tell myself they're just messing around. "You alone?" he continues, and the others laugh, a too-loud laugh that tells me they've been drinking. I keep my head down, grabbing the rest of my stuff and locking the trunk. As I stride toward the side entrance of the hotel, the one closest to my car, the man breaks away from the group and swaggers toward me. I quicken my pace, the warning bells in my head clanging louder. *Almost there,* I tell myself, but when I reach the entrance, the door won't budge. As I jiggle the handle I realize it's one of those doors with a magnetic lock that you have to swipe your room key across to open. I can hear the sound of the man's footsteps approaching, and when I look up his bloated, beery face twists into a sneer.

"Hey baby," he coos, openly appraising my body. "Don't be scared." Panic overtakes me and makes my movements clumsy as I root through my bag, accidentally spilling some of its contents onto the pavement. As I crouch to the ground, scrambling to find my key, an elderly couple appears on the other side of the door. When they push it open, the man steps back, receding into the shadows of the parking lot. I grab my bag and duck into the corridor, the hair on my arms bristling.

Back in the safety of my room, with the door locked and deadbolted behind me, my heart banging hard against my chest, I tell myself to get a grip. I try to remember why it is I've come to this godforsaken place, reminding myself that Lil' GQ had been at the top of my list of people I wanted to visit. To contact him, I'd had to create an online account through a company that allows you to buy digital stamps and to send letters electronically to inmates anywhere in the country. At the time, I didn't know if Lil' GQ would remember me, or if he was still on death row. Each day in the weeks leading up to my departure, I remember eagerly checking my email, hoping for a response. After two weeks of radio silence, I sent a follow-up note through the company's website, but received no reply. I had pretty much given up on hearing from him when it dawned on me: I had failed to include a return address, ignorantly assuming that because I could send Lil' GQ electronic messages, he could send them back, which of course he couldn't, since he wasn't allowed access to a computer.

When I wrote a third time, explaining to Lil' GQ how to reach me, he mailed me a letter right away, saying he was thrilled to learn that I'd survived, and thrilled at the prospect of meeting in person. *To say that I was surprised to hear from you is a true understatement. To be honest with you, I had forgotten about that letter that I wrote to you because I just figured you read it and threw it away.* Lil' GQ asked if we could continue to correspond leading up to our visit so that we might better get to know each other. Since I was making up much of my itinerary on the fly, we had to get creative to keep in touch. I asked him to mail all letters to my parents' address in Saratoga. My parents, in turn, scanned his letters and sent them to me by email. It wasn't the most efficient system, but it worked. By the time I arrived in Livingston, we'd managed to exchange more than a dozen letters.

Stretching out on the bed, I begin skimming the stack of letters in anticipation of our visit, now only a sunrise away. Lil' GQ had been an excellent pen pal: earnest, funny, quick to respond. He'd had a lot of practice, cultivating correspondences with dozens of people over the years. He said it gave him something to do, something to look forward to when the prison guards came around on "mail call" each night. *I enjoy writing letters and learning new things from other folks who've done way more than I have. You see, I've been locked up ever since I was 20 years old and I'm a high school dropout.* The epistolary form, he confessed, also served a practical purpose: *I stutter so writing letters allows me to express myself without feeling insecure and pissed off when I'm having a hard time saying what I want to say.*

Lil' GQ wrote to me about all kinds of things. He wrote to me about his hobbies: *Books are a solitary confinement prisoner's best friend.* He told me about his first car, a stolen brown Cadillac: *I used to get up early in the morning and sit on the hood of my car and watch the projects come alive.* For breast cancer awareness month, he sent me a handmade card with a pink ribbon drawn on it that said: *Courage! Survivor! Friendship! Warrior! Strength!* Lil' GQ's tone was cheerful for the most part, but at times I could sense that he was writing from a defeated place: *Life around here has been the same ole routine for a brotha.* He admitted it was difficult to find the motivation to keep going on certain days, but he was always careful to steer clear of self-pity: *I know that there's a lot of folks who'd love to have as much free time on their hands as I do, just under a different set of circumstances.*

Lil' GQ was thirty-six now, and had spent almost half his life on death row. A lot had changed "out there," he knew, and he was insistent that I tell him all about the world. I did my best to send him updates on my travels. I wrote to him from a Motel 6 in rural Iowa. I wrote to him by the fireplace of a mid-century modern mansion in Jackson, Wyoming. I wrote to him after speaking to a class of eighth graders at a public school in Chicago. The students had written poems inspired by the prompt "where I'm from," and when I shared this with Lil' GQ, he took a stab at his own poem: *I'm from where you didn't always feel a lot of love in the house-*

hold. I'm from where you see nothing but gang members, drug dealers and addicts everywhere. I'm from where you are always being told that a hardhead is a soft behind.

As I got closer to Texas, Lil' GQ put me on his visitation list and filled me in on the rules: Visiting hours would be from 8:00 A.M. to 3:00 P.M. It would be a noncontact visit, meaning we would have to sit on opposite sides of a plexiglass divider and speak to each other through telephone receivers. When I asked if I could bring Lil' GQ books or anything else that he might need, he responded: *Your time and presence is good enough for me. I can look at it as an early Christmas present.*

Hooting and hollering outside the window interrupts my reading. I set the stack of letters down on the bed and stand up. Peeling open the curtains, I spot the group of men from earlier. They've migrated from the recesses of the parking lot to my car, and two of them take a seat on its back bumper as the others stand around clustered in a half circle. I watch as the ringleader of the group, the same guy who came after me, lets out a drunken roar as he pours the dregs of a forty of beer over his head and then smashes the bottle against the pavement. Uneasy, I pick up the room phone and dial reception, explaining the situation. A few minutes later, I see a security guard stroll over. I can't hear what he says, but within minutes, everyone scatters.

Closing the curtains tight, I turn off the lights and climb under the covers. I'm nursing yet another cold and it's hard to fall asleep when I can't breathe so I stand up and root through my duffel bag, searching for a bottle of leftover NyQuil. I take a couple swigs and pull the comforter over my head, my thoughts soon growing sluggish. I don't know how long I'm out, but I'm awakened in the middle of the night by a dull, repetitive sound bludgeoning through my dreams. I groan and roll over onto my stomach, pulling a pil-

low over my head. The sound stops for a moment. Then I hear it
again—*Bam. Bam. Bam.*—like a fusillade. I sit up with a start,
and Oscar leaps off the bed, growling and barking. Without my
contact lenses I can't see anything and I blindly fumble after him
in the dark. The sound appears to be coming from behind my
hotel room door.

"Open up," a man says on the other side. "Open. The. Fucking.
Door." I recognize the voice from somewhere, the slurred speech,
and a shudder ripples through me as I realize it belongs to the man
from the parking lot. Scooping Oscar into my arms, I muzzle his
snout, trying to mute his growls.

"OPEN THE DOOR. IF YOU DON'T OPEN THE FUCK-
ING DOOR . . ." For the first time since I've been on the road, I
feel in acute danger. I know all too well that it takes only one bad
night or one bad-news bearer to revise the way we remember everything that happens before and after. The man slams his fist so
hard against the door that it rattles, his voice growing louder, angrier. Cowering behind the door, my whole body shaking, my
brain tries frantically to make sense of what is happening. The
man must know that I was the one who called hotel security on
him and his friends. Maybe I got them in trouble. That's why he's
so angry. My thoughts go to the small red can of pepper spray I
have tucked away somewhere, but I can't remember if I brought it
in from the car. I want to believe that if this man somehow man-
ages to break in, I will be able to fight him off if I have to, but I
can't seem to move my limbs, much less think straight.

"PABLO! OPEN THE DOOR. OPEN THE MOTHERFUCK-
ING DOOR, PABLO!" the man shouts, and it's only then that I
understand. This man hasn't come for me, he is looking for one of
his friends—he is looking for a man named Pablo, and in his alco-
holic stupor he's mistakenly arrived at my door. With a final, furious bang of his fist, he gives up. I watch through the peephole as
he staggers down the hallway. I stand there for a long while. *Every-*

thing is okay, I tell myself, hugging Oscar tightly against my chest. *I am okay. I am safe. He is gone now.* But no matter what reassurances I whisper to myself, I can't seem to stop shaking.

I've been traveling alone for nearly three months, sleeping in campgrounds and truck stop parking lots, staying at the homes of Internet acquaintances, and crashing with strangers I have met along the way. At every turn, the world has opened its arms to me and treated me with nothing but kindness. The road trip has rekindled a sense of strength and independence I thought I'd never recover, and it wouldn't be an exaggeration to say that it's reaffirmed my trust in humanity. In the last weeks, I've felt clearer, braver, more open to the unknown than I've ever felt in my life. But tonight, I realize that I've also been fortunate. It's something I can't stop thinking about as I return to bed.

The Allan B. Polunsky Unit is the notorious, all-male facility where Texas's death row inmates are housed. Located five miles outside of Livingston, in a heavily forested area known as the Piney Woods, it isn't the kind of place you stumble across by accident. Turning left off the highway, I follow my GPS through farmland, passing a mobile home park, a handful of churches, and fields of horses and abandoned cars under a flat, gray sky.

As I approach the prison's entrance, I see chain-link fence topped with concertina wire, and beyond that a regiment of squat concrete buildings with hundreds of tiny slit windows. Somewhere, behind one of these windows, Lil' GQ is in his cell, preparing for our visit. I roll up to a guard's hut, where a uniformed man circles my car and raps his knuckles against the window, motioning for me to roll it down. "Inmate ID number?" he asks.

I don't have Lil' GQ's ID number memorized, nor do I have it written down, my first of many missteps that day. The guard tells me not to worry and offers to look it up himself. "You drive here all the way from New York?" he asks, examining my driver's license.

I nod.

"Now, that's commitment!" he whistles. "You must be visiting somebody real special."

"You could say that," I reply.

"I went to New York City once. I did my military service in Germany in the seventies and passed through the airport. I didn't like it much. I'm a country boy. You from the Big Apple originally?"

"Yes indeed," I say, nodding.

"You seem like way too nice a young lady to be a New Yorker. Well, there it is. A nice New Yorker and a nice Texan. Who woulda thought?"

The guard assigns me a parking spot in the nearby lot and wishes me a Merry Christmas. I am heartened by our exchange, but once inside the prison I can't seem to do anything right. As soon as I set foot into the main building, a lady in a uniform with bright red hair coiled into a topknot stops me. "You can't bring all that stuff in here," she says, pointing to the pen, notebook, driver's license, and car keys I'm carrying. "Everything needs to go in a clear baggie. You got one?" I shake my head. She motions for me to follow her and we march back out to the parking lot where she pops open the trunk of her car, pulling out an industrial-sized box of clear plastic bags. "We here at the Texas Department of Criminal Justice keep Ziploc in business."

Back inside the prison, I fill out a couple of forms and I am buzzed through a maze of barred doors, leading to the visitation area. As I enter, I am met by a third guard, who takes my visitor's pass and looks me up and down, her gaze narrowing at the sight of my Ziploc bag. "What do you have there?" she asks in a slightly accusatory tone. "You're not supposed to have pen or paper."

"No one told me that," I stammer.

"If it happens again, you'll be banned from visiting," she says sternly, and confiscates them. "Take a seat in R28. The inmate will be brought out soon."

Feeling rattled by our exchange, I enter a room with dozens of white stalls resembling phone booths. By the door, there is a plastic tree decorated in ornaments and a small play area with a rocking horse and a couple of toys, which look out of place here and somehow render the setting even more bleak. I make my way to R28 and take a seat. There's a phone receiver to my left and plexiglass in front of me, just like Lil' GQ described in his letter. On the other side of the plexiglass is a cage-like booth and a stool where, I presume, he will sit. The stalls offer little privacy, and as I wait, I overhear murmurs of conversation. To my left sit three young children, talking shyly to their father. To my right is a graying couple revisiting favorite Christmas carols with their son. *"Feliz Navidad, prospero año y felicidad,"* they sing softly to him through a receiver.

I've been waiting for nearly forty-five minutes when, on the other side of the plexiglass wall, a door clanks open. Lil' GQ walks in. He gives me a jittery grin as a guard unshackles his hand and ankle cuffs. He's shorter than I expected, about my height—five feet seven—handsome with a fresh number two fade. He wears a white short-sleeve prison jumpsuit exposing muscular arms covered in tattoos. As a guard locks the door shut behind him, Lil' GQ takes a seat and picks up the receiver. "I s-s-stutter when I get nervous, and I'm real n-n-nervous right now, so I apologize in advance if that keeps happening," he says.

"I'm also pretty nervous," I admit, which seems to put him at ease. "So, I've been meaning to ask you, what does Lil' GQ stand for anyway?"

"Black people all got nicknames, and mine's short for Gangsta Quin. You got one?"

"Susu. That's what they called me growing up because nobody knew how to pronounce my real name."

"Susu," he says, meeting my eyes for the first time. "I like that. Well, Susu, before we get started with this visit real good, I wanted to thank you for taking the time to come here. It's been about a decade since anybody's visited me, and I've been counting down the days. For real."

Over the next few hours, Lil' GQ begins to tell me all about his life, anecdotes and memories tumbling out of his mouth as though I am a confessor and it is the last time he'll ever tell his story. He tells me about his siblings, four out of five of whom have also been locked up at various points. He tells me about his mother, who was the first person to pull a gun on him: "There wasn't a lot of love shared between us." He tells me about the public housing project where he lived, and about "Agg Land," a neighborhood on Fort Worth's Southside that he repped. With his eyes downcast, he tells me about the relative who molested him starting in elementary school, and how nobody believed him when he spoke up about it. "It was then that I knew that if I wanted to survive in this world I was going to need to learn to fight for myself," he says.

Pressing his forearm against the plexiglass, Lil' GQ shows off a gnarly scar, a welt of puckered skin in the shape of the letter C— C as in Crip, the notorious street gang, he clarifies. He tells me about how, from as early as kindergarten, he knew that's what he wanted to be when he grew up: "Gang members command the most respect in the hood." He tells me about how, at twelve years old, he heated the wire hook of a hanger over a stovetop flame to brand his own flesh as a pledge of loyalty. He shows me another scar, this one on his hand, from the time he fired a bullet clean through his palm on a dare, to the cheers of other gang members. He says he wanted to prove he was a badass despite his age and scrawny frame.

"What makes a badass a badass?" I ask.

He answers with one word: "Violence."

When the guards aren't looking, Lil' GQ unbuttons the front of his jumpsuit to show me a whole story map of scars and tattoos and burn marks on his chest. He tells me about another self-

inflicted gunshot wound, this one on his rib cage. But in this account, there are no cheering bystanders. Instead of becoming the
revered gangster he'd imagined, by the time he was fifteen, he'd
turned into what he described as "the lowest of life-forms inhabit-
ing the hood"—a drug dealer turned drug addict, siphoning from
the supply. One day, while walking alone down the street, he took
out his gun, aimed it at his own chest and pulled the trigger. He
woke up in the emergency room, as his wound was being sutured.

"Why'd you do it?" I ask.

"When you're abused by someone you trust, it confuses you.
When you stay confused, you start to hate yourself." He falls silent
for a minute, a cloud passing over his face.

This seems as good a time as any to ask him about what landed
him here. Lil' GQ tells me point-blank that the murder he is on
death row for isn't the only one he's committed. "I don't feel bad
about those other murders because they were gang-related," he
says. "When you're from where I'm from, the law of the jungle
goes like this: If you don't shoot, they shoot. That's just the way it
is. As for that last murder, the one they got me for, that was messed
up because it was a person I loved. I was high on drugs and needed
more. But I don't blame what I did on the drugs. It was my fault
and for a long time I believed I deserved the death penalty."

I don't know how much of what Lil' GQ is telling me is true.
I'm not searching for holes and inconsistencies, contradictions
and repetitions; I'm just listening. This man has already been
judged for what he has done, and that's not why I came here, anyway. And so I nod, and occasionally I pipe in with a question or an
"I hear that," but mostly I listen. I can't pretend to understand
much about his reality, but the fact that Lil' GQ has a need to share
all of these stories and is trying to make sense of the things that
have happened to him, even now, even on death row, is something
I can understand. When you are forced to confront your mortality,
whether it's because of a diagnosis or a state-mandated death sentence, there's an urgency to lay claim to your life, to shape your

legacy on your own terms, in your own words. To tell stories about your life is to refuse to be reduced to flat inevitability. As I sit here, listening to Lil' GQ talk, I'm reminded of that Joan Didion line: "We tell ourselves stories in order to live." Except that in the case of Lil' GQ, he is telling himself stories in order to ease the passage of death.

"How many appeals do you have left?" I ask.

"One more," he says. A vein pulses in his forehead as he explains the process that leads up to execution. The legal notice that is delivered to your cell, notifying you that a date has been set. The special unit where inmates are transferred in the sixty days before execution and kept under 24/7 surveillance because there are so many suicide attempts. "Some people ask their family to be there when they get executed, but not me. I want to be remembered like *this,* not lying strapped to some table and put down like a dog. Nobody needs that image in their head. I came into this world alone and I'm gonna leave it alone."

When I return the next morning, I come prepared. I have Lil' GQ's inmate ID number written down on a Post-it note, a clear plastic baggie for my wallet, and twenty dollars in coins for the vending machines in case I need a snack. I navigate the labyrinth of hallways and checkpoints, and to my relief, I manage not to get yelled at by any guards. All seems to be going smoothly until Lil' GQ appears on the other side of the greasy plexiglass divider. He looks distraught and I notice puffy bags under his eyes that weren't there yesterday.

"How you feeling?" I ask.

"Honestly? I didn't sleep," he tells me, fidgeting with the cord of the receiver. "I was so nervous yesterday that I started running my mouth like a fool, trying to impress you and whatnot. When you left, I thought for sure that I'd offended you or that you thought I was some crazy deranged killer," he says. "I told my homey in the cell next door that I was sure you weren't coming back. I stayed up all night writing down my thoughts and organizing them so that I'd be able to better express myself in case you did."

Lil' GQ bends over and reaches into his shoe. He pulls out a piece of paper folded into a tiny square. As he opens it, I see that it's covered with notes. He begins to read off a list of questions. He asks about my health and my family. He asks what my favorite book is so that he can read it, too. He asks what breed of dog Oscar is and what kind of music I enjoy. He asks what I did during all that time in the hospital. "I got really, really good at Scrabble," I tell him.

"For real? Me too! I mean, I'm not all that good at Scrabble but I'm trying my hand at it." His whole face lights up as he explains how he and his neighboring prisoners create their own board games out of paper and call out their moves through the vents in the cells where they receive their meal trays. He tells me they're able to play all kinds of games this way, like backgammon and cards.

Lil' GQ says he has never been sick in his life—he does one thousand push-ups each morning to start off the day—but there's a lot about my cancer experience that he relates to. He understands what it's like to feel stuck in purgatory, awaiting the news of your fate; the loneliness and claustrophobia of being confined to a small room for endless stretches of time; how it's necessary to get inventive in order to keep yourself sane. These unexpected parallels are what initially compelled him to write to me. "You've faced death in your own personal prison just like I continue to face death in mine," Lil' GQ says. "At the end of the day death is death, doesn't matter the form it takes."

We are trying so hard to reach through the plexiglass, to meet each other in shared territory we both understand, but what parallels exist between our experiences have their limitations. It's a tricky balance, attempting to find resonance in someone's story without reducing your suffering to sameness. Aside from the obvious differences in skin color and privilege, gender and education, the very fact that I am visiting Lil' GQ while on a road trip underscores an oceanic difference: Mine is a body in motion; his is a body behind bars. But for the duration of our visit we pretend otherwise, both of us acting as if we are in a coffee shop somewhere, just two people chatting away, trying—however imperfectly—to relate to each other.

A tap on my shoulder makes me jump. It's a guard here to tell us it's 3:00 P.M. "My time is up," Lil GQ says. Before I leave, he asks one final question. "If you could take it all back, would you?"

If I could take it all back? I'm stunned. "I don't know," I say, quietly.

These are my last miles. I drive through the bayous of Louisiana, bugs splattering against the windshield. I get caught in a storm on the Alabama coast, run into engine trouble when I forget to change my oil, and stay at an inaptly named Comfort Inn near Daytona Beach, where I wake up to discover I've been bitten all over by fleas. I ring in the New Year with a glorious night of camping on Georgia's Jekyll Island, the sound of waves lulling me to sleep. I stay with an old crush in Charleston, and get slapped with my first-ever speeding ticket, which my mother warns better be my last. Before snaking back up the East Coast, I make a quick stop to cross off one final name on my list: a pint-size teenage girl named Unique, who has spent most of her adolescence living out of hospital rooms, but is now preparing to rejoin the greater gathering. Over lunch, I ask what she wants to do next. She beams at me from across the table with a smile so bright it feels like basking in direct sunlight: "I wanna go to college! And travel! And eat weird foods like octopus that I've never tasted! And come visit you in New York! And go camping, but I'm scared of bugs but I still wanna go camping!" Maybe it's her optimism; maybe it's the long drive over; maybe it's the knowledge that my time on the road is nearly done—

but as I pop a salty fry into my mouth, I think to myself that it is the most delicious fry I've ever tasted.

As I drive on, I continue to ponder Lil' GQ's question. I picture Will, arriving at my doorstep in Paris, both of us so innocent and brimming with hope. I remember my mother's ravaged face as the doctor announced my diagnosis and my father's bloodshot eyes whenever he returned from his walks in the woods. I think back to my brother's faltering grades senior year, the pressure he felt as my donor, the way his needs were constantly overshadowed by mine. In the stillness before sleep, I hear echoes: those quiet moans of suffering, the animal bellows of grief. Of course, I would do anything in my power to spare my loved ones of all pain and terror and heartsickness. Of course, it would have been easier if I had never fallen ill.

Then, my thoughts turn to all the words composed from bed, the letters received, the unexpected friendships made. At a stoplight, I reach back to stroke Oscar, asleep on the backseat. I think of Max, of Melissa—and all those whom I would never have met if it weren't for the loneliness of hospital rooms and the malignant cells that yoked us together. I retrace the distance I've traveled in the last three months—the reckonings and highways and campgrounds. I see Ned, Cecelia, Howard, Nitasha, Bret, Salsa, Katherine, and all the others who have pushed me to plumb new depths. I hear the redwoods' high-up branches creaking in the cool ocean air, the squawking of a fat russet hen being chased around and around a barn, the wind's howl over the plains of Pine Ridge, and the satisfying crunch of pinecones beneath my boots as I pitched my tent for the first time.

Although my twenties have been wrenching, confusing, difficult—to the point of sometimes feeling unendurably painful—they have also been the most formative years of my life, a time imbued with the sweet grace of a second chance, and an inundation of luck, if such a concept can be said to exist at all. The tangling of so much cruelty and beauty has made of my life a strange, discordant landscape. It has left me with an awareness that haunts the edges of my vision—*it can all be lost in a moment*—but it's also given me a jeweler's eye.

If I'm thinking about my illness—abstracted from its impact on the people around me—then the answer is: No, I would not reverse my diagnosis if I could. I would not take back what I suffered to gain this.

EPILOGUE

LIFE IS NOT a controlled experiment. You can't time-stamp when one thing turns into another, can't quantify who impacts you in what way, can't isolate which combination of factors alchemize into healing. There is no atlas charting that lonely, moonless stretch of highway between where you start and who you become. But by the time New York looms into view, the city's mad, glittering skyline blotting out the stars, something in me has shifted, maybe even on a molecular level.

As I cross the George Washington Bridge, my head is full of dreams. Even if I can't see their shapes clearly, or put words to them yet, there are some things I can already make out ahead. I drop off the car, visit my doctor, and move to the little log cabin in Vermont, where I live for several months and begin writing these pages. I read by the fire, wander in the woods, and sit on the back porch. It's there on this porch, on an afternoon later that summer, that I receive the news that Max has died. *"Heaven,"* he wrote in one of his last poems,

is really just a hospital for souls.
When I get there, I will get there
and it will not be complicated

I am not that sick in Heaven.

Whenever I wake up missing my friends, I visit them through their words and watercolors.

My immune system keeps misfiring. I still push my body too hard. I am hospitalized for complications of the flu that turn into sepsis. I am forced to accept my limitations and slowness—a lesson I must learn again and again. I get discouraged. I stop writing these pages. I rest, recover, begin again.

It takes a good while longer, and a couple more detours, but Jon and I eventually make a real go of things. We move to a quiet, tree-lined block in Brooklyn. On our first night there, we celebrate, eating takeout by candlelight amid piles of moving boxes. I unpack my double bass, dust it off for the first time in years, and Jon warms up the piano. Together, we begin to play.

My brother, now a fourth-grade teacher, lives in my old apartment in the East Village and has repainted the walls with his own stories and memories and heartbreaks. My parents relocate to Tunisia temporarily, and I return to visit for the first time since college. I eat my aunt Fatima's famous couscous, spend time with my cousins, and celebrate the New Year in the Sahara. My father is getting ready to retire and when he does, he plans on embarking upon a cross-country road trip of his own, following my same itinerary. My mother, no longer a full-time parent or caregiver, has turned her energies back to painting and has resumed her career as an artist, attaining successes and a sense of agency that she assumed had been foreclosed long ago.

There are certain dreams I can't dream, for I never thought them possible. The week after my thirtieth birthday, I complete a half marathon. I return to Ojai, where I spend three months as a visiting teacher at Katherine's school. Inspired by the experience of meeting Lil' GQ, I write my first reported feature, not from bed, but from the field, about a prison hospice in Northern California. One afternoon, while procrastinating on these pages, I come across a "for sale" ad for a 1972 Volkswagen camper van the color of Sunshine. I write to the owner, a retired U.S. Air Force officer, who it turns out is receiving treatment at Sloan Kettering and recognizes my name from my *New York Times* columns written all those years ago. "Name a price and she's yours," he says. "Nobody ever bought one of these old ladies to be practical."

I keep the van at the cabin in Vermont and attempt to learn how to drive a stick shift. I fumble with the gears and pound the steering wheel in frustration as I stall out too many times to count. Jerking along the back roads near the cabin, I shift from first to second gear, the engine spluttering and whining as I drive up to the top of a nearby mountain still dusted in snow. As I reach the summit, the road turns smooth and flat. Cruising along a dirt path, I pick up speed, passing evergreens fanged with ice. Oscar sits in the passenger's seat, watching the trees blur past. In the icebox I've packed a smoked chicken, a bottle of wine, and a book. It's been a while since we've been able to get away, and for the next few days, it's just the two of us. Wherever I am, wherever we go, home will always be the in-between place, a wilderness I've grown to love.

ACKNOWLEDGMENTS

To Richard Pine, king among agents, and Carrie Cook, who helped me turn a bar napkin into a book—I am endlessly grateful. To my editor, Andy Ward, for his enormous care, kindness, and guidance, and to the late legendary Susan Kamil, for believing from the beginning. To my old pal and assistant editor, Sam Nicholson, and to the many other wonderful people at Penguin Random House: in particular, Marie Pantojan, Susan Mercandetti, Carrie Neill, and Paolo Pepe, as well as my foreign editors, especially Andrea Henry. Special thanks to Ben Phelan, who shouldered the challenging task of fact-checking this book, and did so with unparalleled sensitivity, compassion, and good humor.

A great debt is owed to Lizzie Presser, my dearest friend, who always reads first and who championed this book long before I had the confidence to write it. To Carmen Radley, brilliant quarantine comrade, writer, and reader, who ushered me to the end. To the matchless Lindsay Ryan, who made these pages immeasurably better, and to Vrinda Condillac, who saw what was needed and helped me untangle the threads. And many thanks to early readers and to my mentors: Glenn Brown, Lisa Ann Cockrel, Chris McCormick, Jenny Boully, Peter Trachtenberg, Esmé Weijun Wang, Lily Brooks-Dalton, Katherine Halsey, and Bonnie Davidson. To my writing group for being stellar company during this sometimes lonely, always arduous endeavor: Jordan Kisner, Jayson Greene, Frank Scott, and especially Melissa Febos and Tara Westover, who offered invaluable advice.

For the gift of time and quiet when it was most needed, I am grateful to the Ucross Foundation, Kerouac Project, New York Public Library, Anacapa Fellowship, and Stone Acres Farm, as well as to the cabin in Vermont, where many of these words were written. To the Bennington Writing Seminars, for providing a beloved community. Deep thanks to Christina Merrill for her exceeding generosity, to Gideon Irving for entrusting me with his car, and to the Presser, Nelson-Greenberg, and Ross families for gifting me haven and support when I needed it most. My thanks also to Erin Allweiss, Marissa Mullen, Lindsay Ratowsky, and Maya Land, for their tireless efforts behind the scenes.

A last, deep bow to those who make my world possible: To my parents—my deepest love and most profound thanks—and to my brother, Adam, for quite literally saving my life. To Dr. Holland, Dr. Navada, Dr. Silverman, Dr. Castro, and Dr. Liebers, and to my nurses Alli Tucker, Abbie Cohen, Sunny, and Younique, as well as the countless other healthcare professionals, for without them, I wouldn't be here. To Jon Batiste, who taught me to believe again and who braved with grace and patience the long stretches I had to be away. To Tara Parker-Pope, who gave me my first break, and to my professor Marty Gottlieb, for the introduction. To Mara, Natalie, Kristen, Erika, Michelle, Lilli, Behida, Ruthie, Azita, Kate, Sylvie, and the many other women, too numerous to name here, who lift me up with their friendship. And, finally, to my road guardians, for opening their homes and sharing their stories with me. Thank you for guiding me through the most difficult passage.